W9-AXF-688

OUTBREAK!

50 TALES OF EPIDEMICS THAT TERRORIZED THE WORLD

BETH SKWARECKI

Aadamsmedia

AVON, MASSACHUSETTS

To my children. This is why you have all your shots.

≡≝

Published by
Adams Media, a division of F+W Media, Inc.
57 Littlefield Street, Avon, MA 02322. U.S.A.
www.adamsmedia.com

ISBN 10: 1-4405-9627-1
ISBN 13: 978-1-4405-9627-8
eISBN 10: 1-4405-9628-X
eISBN 13: 978-1-4405-9628-5

Printed in the United States of America.

10 9 8 7 6 5 4 3 2 1

Library of Congress Cataloging-in-Publication Data

Skwarecki, Beth, author.
Outbreak! / Beth Skwarecki.
Avon, Massachusetts: Adams Media, [2016]
LCCN 2016015141 (print) | LCCN 2016024010 (ebook) | ISBN 9781440596278 (pb) |
ISBN 1440596271 (pb) | ISBN 9781440596285 (ebook) | ISBN 144059628X (ebook)
LCSH: Epidemics--History. | BISAC: MEDICAL / History. | HEALTH & FITNESS / Diseases
/ Contagious.
LCC RA649 .S59 2016 (print) | LCC RA649 (ebook) | DDC 614.4--dc23
LC record available at https://lccn.loc.gov/2016015141

Cover design by Stephanie Hannus.
Cover and interior images © Clipart.com, iStockphoto.com/Roberto A Sanchez.

This book is available at quantity discounts for bulk purchases.
For information, please call 1-800-289-0963.

CONTENTS

7   INTRODUCTION

9   CHAPTER 1
World Takeover: Malaria   • 10,000 B.C.E.
Africa

13   CHAPTER 2
The Fiery Serpent: Guinea Worm   • 1495 B.C.E.
Red Sea

18   CHAPTER 3
The Plague of Athens: Unknown Disease   • 430 B.C.E.
Athens

23   CHAPTER 4
Galen's Plague: Smallpox   • C.E. 165
Rome

28   CHAPTER 5
The Plague of Justinian: Bubonic Plague   • C.E. 542
Constantinople

32   CHAPTER 6
A Vicious Cycle: Smallpox   • C.E. 735
Japan

37   CHAPTER 7
Message from a Sacred Mountain: Smallpox   • C. 1000
China

41   CHAPTER 8
Saint Anthony's Fire: Ergotism   • 1095
France

45   CHAPTER 9
A Doomed Crusade: Scurvy   • 1249
Egypt

49   CHAPTER 10
The Knights of Lazarus: Leprosy (Hansen's Disease)   • 1200s
Europe

CONTENTS

54   CHAPTER 11
      China's Plague: Bubonic Plague
    c. 1331
    China

59   CHAPTER 12
      The Black Death: Bubonic Plague
    1348
    Europe

64   CHAPTER 13
      The Sweating Sicknes: Unknown Disease
    1485
    England

68   CHAPTER 14
      The First Invaders: Influenza
    1493
    Hispaniola/Haiti

72   CHAPTER 15
      The French Disease: Syphilis
    1495
    Italy

77   CHAPTER 16
      The Dancing Plague: Mass Psychogenic Illness
    1518
    Strasbourg

82   CHAPTER 17
      The Fall of Moctezuma: Smallpox
    1520
    Tenochtitlán

86   CHAPTER 18
      The Lost Cure for Scurvy: Scurvy
    1536
    Stadacona

90   CHAPTER 19
      The King's Evil: Scrofula
    1594
    France

94   CHAPTER 20
      Squanto's Backstory: Unknown Disease
    1616
    Massachusetts

99   CHAPTER 21
      The First Miracle Cure: Malaria
    1630
    Peru

104   CHAPTER 22
      The Great Plague of London: Bubonic Plague
    1665
    London

109   CHAPTER 23
      Scourge of a Young Nation's Capital: Yellow Fever
    1793
    Philadelphia

114   CHAPTER 24
      Peeing Red: Schistosomiasis
    1799
    Egypt

CONTENTS

118   **CHAPTER 25**
The Romantic Disease: Tuberculosis

123   **CHAPTER 26**
The Haitian Revolution: Yellow Fever

127   **CHAPTER 27**
Birth of a Pandemic: Cholera

131   **CHAPTER 28**
Childbed Fever: Uterine Infection

136   **CHAPTER 29**
Mapping Death: Cholera

141   **CHAPTER 30**
Exiled on Molokai: Leprosy (Hansen's Disease)

145   **CHAPTER 31**
Beat of the Death-Drum: Measles

150   **CHAPTER 32**
Tunnel of Anemia: Hookworm

155   **CHAPTER 33**
Rabies Loses Its Bite: Rabies

159   **CHAPTER 34**
The Beriberi Box: Beriberi

164   **CHAPTER 35**
The Chinatown Plague: Bubonic Plague

169   **CHAPTER 36**
Down by the Riverside: Sleeping Sickness

173   **CHAPTER 37**
Typhoid Mary and Friends: Typhoid Fever

178   **CHAPTER 38**
An Unpopular Discovery: Pellagra

1800s
England

1802
Saint-Domingue

1817
India

1847
Vienna

1854
London

1866
Hawaii

1875
Fiji

1880
Switzerland

1885
Paris

1884
Japan

1900
San Francisco

1901
Uganda

1907
New York

1914
Mississippi

CONTENTS

183 CHAPTER 39
The "Spanish" Flu: Influenza
• 1918
Worldwide

187 CHAPTER 40
Serum by Dogsled: Diphtheria
• 1925
Alaska

192 CHAPTER 41
Just Another Horror: Typhus
• 1945
Poland

197 CHAPTER 42
The Beginning of the End for Polio: Polio
• 1952
USA

202 CHAPTER 43
Breakbone Fever: Dengue Hemorrhagic Fever
• 1953
Philippines

207 CHAPTER 44
The Brain-Eating Amoeba:
Primary Amebic Meningoencephalitis
• 1965
Australia

211 CHAPTER 45
The Leak from Compound 19: Anthrax
• 1979
USSR

216 CHAPTER 46
AIDS Panic and Progress: AIDS
• 1980s
USA

221 CHAPTER 47
Mad Cow Spreads to Humans:
Transmissible Spongiform Encephalopathy
• 1996
England

227 CHAPTER 48
The Locker Room Menace: MRSA
• 2002
Los Angeles

231 CHAPTER 49
The Secret Epidemic: SARS
• 2003
Hong Kong

236 CHAPTER 50
Ebola Is Real: Ebola
• 2014
West Africa

242 FURTHER READING

251 INDEX

INTRODUCTION

P lague after plague has swept the earth, many changing the course of history. Armies have been decimated, emperors felled, boats full of warriors turned around on what would have been the eve of battle. We like to think it's people that rule the earth, but germs wield much more power.

Today we are still not completely in control. We can slow pandemics, stop them, make them more rare, but never entirely prevent them. Nature keeps surprising us: Ebola killed more people in 2014 than in all of its previous outbreaks combined. Whole villages were wiped out, leaving nobody to run stores or restaurants or provide ordinary health care for nonlethal ailments. Bodies were collected en masse and buried or cremated with little ceremony and, sometimes, nobody left to grieve.

At least scientists understood the cause, and were able to set to work on the treatments and vaccines that could prevent the next outbreak. That wasn't the case when the Black Death struck Europe. With frightening fierceness, it produced a steady stream of bodies for mass graves, and doctors scrambled for cures. They tried bloodletting, prayer, potions of fermented spices. Instead of plasticky yellow bodysuits, plague doctors wore waxed leather cloaks and gloves, and breathed through masks stuffed with sweet-smelling herbs. Nobody had yet figured out how disease spreads, but avoiding the stench of death and squalor seemed like a good precaution to take.

Before this plague there were others: leprosy, malaria, tuberculosis. Smallpox lesions have been found on mummies. Skeletons thousands of years old show bone deformities that may be syphilis.

With thousands of years of practice in disease fighting, we are finally beginning to get it right. Bubonic plague still exists, but it can be killed by antibiotics. Smallpox, thanks to vaccines, is extinct in the wild. Cholera is a thing of the past in places where drinking water and sewage run in separate pipes. The first vaccine for dengue, the tropical "breakbone fever," has finally made its debut.

This book follows these diseases through history, along with our often ill-fated attempts to understand and treat them. It tells the stories of history's most infamous outbreaks, from ancient scourges to modern-day medical mysteries. We will mourn for the dead, fear for the living, and applaud the helpers who risked their lives to care for the sick. With each century, it seems, we manage to steal a little more power from our foes the germs.

CHAPTER 1

WORLD TAKEOVER

MALARIA: AFRICA

10,000 B.C.E.

ONE OF THE OLDEST DISEASES KNOWN TO HUMANKIND IS STILL RAMPANT TODAY. MALARIA STARTED SMALL, BUT WITH THE HELP OF MOSQUITOES, IT TOOK OVER THE WORLD.

DEATH TOLL: Unknown; millions

CAUSED BY: Mosquito-borne *Plasmodium* parasites

NOTEWORTHY SYMPTOMS: Chills and a fever that recurs every few days

FATALITY RATE: Unknown; today the fatality rate is less than 1 percent

THREAT LEVEL TODAY: High in many parts of the world.

NOTABLE FACT: About 7 percent of people alive today have at least one gene that helps them resist malaria.

L ong, long ago, malaria hit the big time.

You would think this amoeba-like parasite was already doing pretty well, living inside people's red blood cells and scarfing down their life-giving hemoglobin. But at first it was only doing this in a small neighborhood—probably the east coast of Africa, around where Ethiopia is today.

But malaria spread. It covered all of Asia before long, including India and China. It expanded into the Mediterranean, and from there through Europe. The eastern coast of England was once known as a place eager to give visitors malarial fevers.

It's hard to pinpoint the date of this spread, especially because many of the people involved didn't know how to write—or if they did, and they wrote about malaria, their writings may not have survived. But once they figured out how to put ink on papyrus or silk, people around the world began writing about malaria: how to diagnose it and what to do once you've figured out somebody has it. The Chinese *Huang-Ti Nei Ching* (*The Canon of Internal Medicine*), the Indian Atharva Veda, and the writings of Hippocrates in Greece all describe fevers that were probably malaria.

WHAT'S GOING ON IN THERE

Malaria isn't caused by a bacterium or a virus, but by a protozoan. Think of an amoeba, if that helps: a single-celled creature that's related more closely to us than to bacteria, but is still small enough to fit inside one of our cells.

The parasite enters a person's body with a mosquito bite, and rides the bloodstream to the liver to hide until it can make more of itself—amassing an army for its next step, which is a takeover of blood cells.

The liquid part of our blood is clear, and on its own would be unimpressive looking. But it's filled with round red cells that keep us alive. With every heartbeat blood goes to the lungs, where the cells are suddenly surrounded in oxygen. That oxygen sticks to the hemoglobin inside the red blood cells, and with the next heartbeat the cells whoosh on their way.

Traveling to the cells' destination—maybe a muscle, or a vital organ—the oxygen remains stuck to an iron atom in the center of the hemoglobin proteins. The malaria parasite has its figurative eye on that hemoglobin.

When the army of parasites leaves the liver to attack the red blood cells, the body finally realizes it's been invaded, and for the first time, the person is racked with chills and develops a high fever. Many of the parasites are killed, but a few make it into the blood cells, where once again they are protected. The fever subsides. But soon a new batch of parasites bursts out.

The cycles happen when each generation of the parasite has eaten its fill of hemoglobin and bursts out of the blood cells. The body attacks again, causing a new cycle of chills and fever. The pieces of cells float in the bloodstream until the spleen filters them out. The overworked spleen can end up twenty times its normal size.

Each type of malaria has its own pattern, making it easy to recognize from historical texts. *Plasmodium malariae*, a fairly mild version, causes a fever that disappears the next day, only to come back on day four: a quartan fever. *P. vivax*, rare in Africa but common elsewhere, causes fevers that return on the third day. *P. falciparum*, one of the nastiest types of malaria, also works on a three-day cycle; it's called the "malignant tertian."

WRITING ITS STORY

Some diseases are older than written history. Many of them, in fact. We know about yaws, a relative of the notorious sexually transmitted disease syphilis, only because it leaves distinctive marks on bones, and archaeologists have dug up those bones. The same rings true for leprosy: it is present in some ancient bones, so we know the disease must be ancient.

Malaria's history is written not on some old bones, but in DNA. Scientists have calculated that the species of the malaria parasite that infect people today are probably older than the human species itself. Our closest animal cousins, chimpanzees, have their own, closely related malaria parasite. This disease is so dangerous, and knows us so well, that even after half a million years it still takes credit for one of every six child deaths in Africa. Worldwide, that's a child every minute. It's not very kind to adults either.

One early form of the malaria parasite, probably a close relative of the one known today as *Plasmodium vivax*, must have killed enormous numbers of Africans. We know this because *P. vivax* uses a set of proteins, called Duffy proteins, as a doorknob to get into red blood cells. Sometime after the great migrations out of Africa, when people with Duffy proteins were scattered over the globe, somebody in Africa lucked out and was born without Duffy proteins. This person was not susceptible to *P. vivax* malaria. In time this person's lucky children came to populate almost the entire continent.

That's why *P. vivax* is rare in Africa today, although it's common in places like South America and Indonesia. Africa now has to deal with a younger, deadlier version of malaria, *P. falciparum*. There's a gene that helps with this, too. It's a change in the instructions to make hemoglobin, so the hemoglobin itself thwarts the parasite. Children who get one copy of this gene and one of the normal hemoglobin gene are protected against malaria. Children who get a double dose of the special hemoglobin have a blood disorder called sickle cell anemia, which can also be deadly. But in the big picture, malaria is so dangerous that the sickle cell roulette game is worth playing.

In all, one of every fourteen people on earth has some kind of genetic mutation that protects them from malaria—a sign that their ancestors were survivors in a long-ago fight against the disease. These are in some cases the only records we have of long-ago outbreaks that shattered families and decimated villages. Though we now have medicines for malaria we don't yet have a vaccine, and the parasite often becomes resistant to what would otherwise be a cure. Despite the best efforts of modern medicine, malaria is still widespread in the world today.

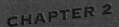

CHAPTER 2

THE FIERY SERPENT

GUINEA WORM: RED SEA

1495 B.C.E.

A WORM THAT BURROWS THROUGH YOUR BODY UNTIL IT CHEWS ITS WAY OUT THROUGH YOUR TOE; CLEARLY THIS IS THE STUFF OF NIGHTMARES.

DEATH TOLL: Unknown

CAUSED BY: The guinea worm, *Dracunculus medinensis*

NOTEWORTHY SYMPTOMS: A burning, painful blister on the foot or leg

FATALITY RATE: Less than 1 percent

THREAT LEVEL TODAY: Low. Thanks to an international effort to prevent the disease, guinea worm disease is expected to go extinct in the near future.

NOTABLE FACT: While you might think pulling the worm out of your body to rid yourself of the nasty thing is a good idea, think again. Pulling and breaking the worm can lead to infections and possible limb loss.

One of the oldest tales of a parasite epidemic is short, sketchy, and leaves some room for interpretation. That's par for the course in ancient history. But to parasitologists, it rings out clearly as a cautionary tale about a worm that causes horrific pain and, if you're not careful, potential death.

The culprit is known today as the guinea worm, but in antiquity it went by names that translate as "little dragon" and "the gnawer from Medina." The Guinea worm resembles a three-foot-long strand of spaghetti, and it eats its way through the body from the inside. Only when it is about to poke its head out of a person's skin does that person begin to feel the itching and burning that signal the beginning of weeks or months of agony.

The Old Testament tells the story like this. Moses and the Israelites had been traveling for years through the desert. On a particularly rough leg of the journey, the people began to complain: "Wherefore have you brought us up out of Egypt to die in the wilderness? For there is no bread, neither is there any water; and our soul loatheth this light bread."

Yahweh doesn't like whiners, it seems, because the next verse simply states that "the Lord sent fiery serpents among the people, and they bit the people; and much people of Israel died." This may, arguably, refer to a "serpent" that burrows from the skin rather than the regular reptilian type that bites.

Whichever it was, we do know that the little dragons plagued people along the Red Sea around that time. The Ebers Papyrus, an Egyptian medical text from 1550 B.C.E., gives instructions for treating a worm embedded in a person's skin. Archaeologists found a calcified guinea worm in a mummified person that died around 1000 B.C.E.

The Israelites are finally saved from the serpents when Moses makes a brass sculpture of a serpent on a pole. This may be an early public health effort, a visual aid to teach the proper treatment for guinea worm. Because when that yard-long piece of spaghetti begins to emerge from the painful, fiery blister it causes, the best course of action—even today—is to wrap the worm around a tiny stick. This keeps it from slinking back into the body. With careful wrapping, over the course of weeks, the fiery serpent can be drawn out and removed.

THE WORM'S JOURNEY

The guinea worm's life cycle begins and ends in shallow ponds, where people wade to collect drinking water. If the area is a desert, which means there are only a few of these ponds, so much the better from the guinea worm's point of view; everyone in the neighborhood will have to come to the watering hole, so the worm has its best chance of transmission.

Guinea worms spend their childhood inside of a water flea, a distant relative of lobsters that is barely the size of the head of a pin. The baby worms wriggle until the water flea eats them, and then they turn the tables. They chew through the water flea's stomach and feast on its ovaries or testes. They bide their time until a human wanders by, collecting drinking water. If there are enough baby worms in a small enough pond, they stand a good chance of being scooped up.

Our digestive system dissolves what's left of the water flea, releasing the worm larvae. They burrow out of our small intestine and into the body at large, burrowing through organs and vessels. Somewhere on her journey, already a few inches long, a lucky female will meet a male. They mate, the male dies, and the female moves on. She burrows downward, following blood vessels and connective tissue, most of the time ending in the foot or leg.

All the while, she is growing. Her vital organs don't take up much space, so the bulk of her three-foot-long body is dedicated to uterus. By the time she is mature, she contains 3 million tiny eggs, which hatch inside of her, creating 3 million baby worms eager to swim into the nearest body of water.

So far the human host has not felt anything unusual. It takes a year, more or less, for the worm to find its way. Normally our immune system would kick out any intruders, but parasitic worms know how to fly under the radar. The host's body doesn't seem to notice the worm until it's almost ready to emerge. Allergic symptoms, like hives and itching, may herald its exit.

A blister forms. Let's say it's on the person's foot, although worms have been known to emerge from hands, eyelids, even genitals. The blister burns and itches and burns and aches, and the only thing that relieves the pain is water. Our sufferer finds a pond to step in: ahh, relief. The water triggers the protruding worm to squirt out a cloud of what looks like milky liquid. It's actually a batch of baby worms, 50,000 or so.

AS THE WORM TURNS

The mother worm won't die until all 3 million of her offspring have been released. That's a lot of trips to the watering hole, over the course of weeks or even months. During this time, the guinea worm sufferer may be in so much pain it's not possible to walk or work. Entire villages become incapacitated during guinea worm season. Children can't walk to school, farmers can't farm, parents can't take care of their children.

Wrapping the worm around a stick, slowly pulling it out, can shorten the infection: at an inch a day, the worm can be removed in a few weeks. The human host may still have a few weeks or months of painful healing ahead, but that's the best-case scenario.

What's worse is pulling hard on the worm and breaking it. The worm dies, but that's no victory. The larvae spill out into the surrounding body parts, and our immune system notices for the first time that a massive worm is embedded in body tissues. It attacks the dying worm and its children, and human tissue often dies as collateral damage. The body part containing the worm is now more susceptible to infection, including cellulitis and gangrene.

Some people survive, but breaking the worm is extremely risky. It's understandable why Hebrew scholar and parasitologist Friedrich Küchenmeister saw the biblical story as an explanation of guinea worm treatment. The Israelites would be new to the guinea worms' home territory, and may have pulled at the worms at first. Breaking the worm could lead to death, but wrapping it could save them.

Today, that's still the best treatment we have. Medicines that kill other worms don't work on guinea worm; they can even make a guinea worm change course and burrow into parts of the body where it's not usually found. But the course of the disease in human history has been changed by simple understanding.

Since the worms enter the body inside pinhead-sized water fleas, a simple filter can defeat the parasite. A scrap of filter cloth over the end of a pipe makes a straw that nomads can use to drink water minus the water fleas. Villages that used to boast a few ponds or a wide well as their water source can wipe out the infection by switching to a type of well that you don't stick your feet into. Methods like this brought infection rates down from 40 million in the middle of the twentieth century to 3.5 million in 1986, when the World Health Organization and the Carter Center began an anti–guinea worm campaign, and to just 22 reported cases in 2015.

If the guinea worm goes extinct, the disease it causes will be gone forever. It will be only the second human disease to be eradicated. (The first was smallpox.) Learning about the worm gave us the means to fight it, but humankind has not been so lucky with other illnesses.

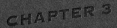

CHAPTER 3

THE PLAGUE OF ATHENS

UNKNOWN DISEASE: ATHENS

430 B.C.E.

THE MYSTERY OF THE UNKNOWN DISEASE THAT RAVAGED THE WALLED CITY OF ATHENS REMAINS UNSOLVED TO THIS DAY. WAS IT A PLAGUE OF THE GODS OR SOMETHING MORE SINISTER?

DEATH TOLL: 75,000 (estimated)

CAUSED BY: Unknown disease; typhoid, measles, smallpox, and Ebola have been suggested

NOTEWORTHY SYMPTOMS: Headache, rash, bloody diarrhea, gangrene of fingers and toes

FATALITY RATE: 25 percent (estimated)

THREAT LEVEL TODAY: Unknown

NOTABLE FACT: This is one of the first epidemics to ever be described in detail in a historical text.

One of the first grisly blow-by-blows of a deadly epidemic comes from the Greek historian Thucydides. It's just one chapter in his chronicle of the Peloponnesian War, but it changed the course of that war and gave medical detectives a mystery to puzzle over for centuries.

At first, Thucydides writes, the young men of Athens were enthusiastic about the war against Sparta and the Peloponnesian League. After a rough first year, the Athenian leader, Pericles, presided over a large public funeral, delivering a stirring speech about the greatness of Athens. But as soon as the speech concludes, Thucydides's tale cuts immediately to the horrors of the following summer's plague.

Despite the name, the disease was probably not related to the bubonic plague, which would strike the area centuries later. This plague, this epidemic, produced symptoms that have never been nailed down to a specific cause. The Athenians didn't recognize it either, and their doctors found all the usual cures to be useless. At first they thought the enemy might have poisoned their water.

"People in good health were all of a sudden attacked by violent heats in the head," Thucydides begins, and he traces the path of the disease on an orderly march through the body.

The eyes became red and inflamed, and then there was bleeding from the tongue and throat. After that came respiratory symptoms, including sneezing and cough, and then the afflicted would vomit bile. Next came a symptom that is sometimes translated as retching, but might have been hiccups.

Meanwhile, the skin broke out in a rash, with "small pustules and ulcers." The affected skin was so sensitive that the sufferers could not wear clothes, and wanted to cool themselves in water. If they survived long enough, the historian wrote, they would suffer bloody diarrhea. People would lose their fingers, toes, and "privy parts," and survivors would sometimes find they had lost their memory.

THE WAR

The epidemic played out within the walls of the city of Athens. The Athenians' military strategy was an odd one: when the Peloponnesians attacked, the Athenians did not fight, but instead invited the people of the surrounding countryside to live within the city walls. Those walls extended to the southwest to include the port of Piraeus. Athens had a strong navy, and the city's leaders banked on their warships' ability to get supplies to and from the port.

After just forty days, the Peloponnesians gave up the siege, possibly because they noticed the funeral pyres and decided they wanted nothing to do with a city where disease was raging. Inside the city, Thucydides writes, people were hopeless. Sufferers died whether anybody took care of them or not, so neighbors and families faced the dilemma of abandoning their loved ones or caring for them knowing that they too would soon be sick.

Temple offerings were just as useless as doctors' treatment; the plague went on. Maybe, some of the people whispered, the gods have forsaken us. The plague went on for years, and returned multiple times. Survivors emerged as heroes, because after they recovered they were immune to the disease and were not afraid to nurse the sick. Their experience helped them comfort the afflicted, since they understood the course of the disease. This isn't a medical account, some scholars have argued, but a story about morality. The people who cared for the sick stand in contrast to those who chose to enjoy life while they could, frittering away money they couldn't take with them, breaking the law because they believed they wouldn't live to stand trial.

THE DISEASE

We still don't know, and may never know, what disease caused the Plague of Athens. But if the symptoms are accurately described, as Thucydides insists they are, it should be possible to compare them to known viruses and bacteria and come up with a good guess.

Bubonic plague is unlikely. Thucydides does not describe the disease's signature swollen lymph nodes, or buboes, and bubonic plague has no rash or diarrhea. Smallpox might fit the description of the rash, depending on whether "pustules" is the right translation for the word he used. If instead the rash was flat on the skin, the disease could be measles. Typhus, carried by lice and known throughout history for its association with armies, is another front-runner.

There is one more theory, strengthened in recent years. The symptoms of the Plague of Athens match fairly well to hemorrhagic fevers, especially Ebola. Ebola's symptoms include fever and headache, vomiting and diarrhea, eye inflammation, and any of a variety of skin rashes. Hiccups are a notable symptom. As in Thucydides's time, the disease passes easily to doctors and caregivers, and survivors are immune to further infection.

When the Ebola theory was first proposed in the 1990s, it seemed weak; Ebola outbreaks never lasted more than a few months, and it wasn't realistic to expect a person or animal to carry the virus all the way from Africa. Those assumptions turned out to be wrong: In 2014, Ebola somehow traveled thousands of miles and even with an international response, the outbreak lasted for more than a year.

In 1994, archaeologists found a burial pit near the ancient Kerameikos cemetery in Athens. Vases in the grave date it to the time of the epidemic. Bodies were laid down haphazardly in what became the bottom layer, and then more bodies were packed closer together and apparently with less care in the layers that came later.

Researchers extracted teeth from some of the skeletons. Teeth have blood vessels inside them, so any bacteria in the bloodstream would be preserved there, and germs from the outside would be unlikely to find their way inside the tooth. DNA analysis showed that the teeth contained the bacterium responsible for typhoid fever (no relation to typhus). The researchers also tested for bubonic plague, anthrax, and tuberculosis, among others, and found no matches.

But was typhoid fever really the cause of death? Some of the symptoms match, but typhoid's rash isn't quite right, survivors don't become immune, and the disease has a low mortality rate. Maybe they had typhoid *plus* Ebola, or some other disease. If that's the case, it will probably remain a mystery. Some viruses, including Ebola and measles, carry their genes in RNA, not DNA, and RNA is less likely to last through centuries. If the cause was one of these viruses, we may never find a smoking gun.

CHAPTER 4

GALEN'S PLAGUE

SMALLPOX: ROME

C.E. 165

THIS PLAGUE MAY HAVE BROUGHT DOWN THE ROMAN EMPIRE, DESPITE THE EFFORTS OF THE BIGGEST CELEBRITY DOCTOR OF THE TIME: GALEN OF PERGAMON.

DEATH TOLL: Unknown; possibly 5 million

CAUSED BY: Probably the smallpox virus *Variola major*

NOTEWORTHY SYMPTOMS: A rash of pustules

FATALITY RATE: 25 percent

THREAT LEVEL TODAY: Gone. Smallpox has been eradicated through worldwide vaccination.

NOTABLE FACT: Galen's ideas (many now understood to be false) would underlie medical treatments for more than a millennium—including the way doctors approached many of the plagues that followed.

Roman soldiers were far from Rome when they attacked two cities on the Tigris River in what today is Iraq. First they invaded Ctesiphon, on the left side of the river, and burned the royal palace. Across the water, the city of Seleucia opened its gates in surrender. The Romans sacked the city anyway.

The soldiers made a fateful mistake, according to legend, when they ransacked a temple dedicated to the god Apollo. Apollo looked down from Mount Olympus and cursed a treasure chest that the men carried away. When they opened the chest, they found it full of not riches but pestilence. The plague—legend or not—really did sweep the entire Roman kingdom. It raged for decades, devastated the kingdom, and probably killed at least one emperor. Such is the wrath of the gods. Or, you know, smallpox.

We don't have a single clear account of the plague and its symptoms, but Galen of Pergamon scattered descriptions and remedies throughout his voluminous writings. He treated soldiers who suffered from the plague and even treated the emperor, Marcus Aurelius. But the plague barely rates as a highlight in Galen's career. His medical texts ended up as the core of medical education for more than a millennium afterward—even though many of his ideas were utterly wrong.

GALEN, CELEBRITY DOCTOR

Say you were a patent-medicine huckster and you wanted to sell your special medicine that could get rid of worms in people's teeth. You announce this in front of a crowd, and if you say you got this medicine from Galen, people will listen. Here is where you bring up a volunteer, blow medicinal smoke in his face, and while his eyes are closed you slip worms into his mouth and then pretend to pull them out.

Galen wrote about being in the crowd when a charlatan pulled this exact stunt. He revealed himself to the crowd, shouting, "I am Galen, and he is a swindler!" He then turned in the huckster to local authorities to be flogged.

Despite his fame, Galen's treatments for diseases like the plague probably weren't any better than the charlatan's. Doctors of the day were stumped by many illnesses, and were far away from figuring out how the body works. That didn't stop Galen or other ancient writers from arguing over the body's workings. Galen dissected dead animals, and even experimented cruelly on living ones, to figure out the functions of body parts. For example, it was news when he revealed that arteries contain blood and not air.

Being doctor to the gladiators probably also gave him a window into anatomy—literally, in the gladiators' wounds. Galen wrote anatomical texts that lived on for more than a thousand years before Andreas Vesalius, in 1543, dissected people instead of animals and discovered some of Galen's errors.

Wounds and anatomy are simple, in a sense: you can see whatever body parts are in front of your eyes. But diseases are more subtle. What causes a fever, or a cold? Galen, borrowing from Hippocrates, wrote ferocious defenses of the then-controversial theory of the four humors.

Blood, phlegm, yellow bile, and an imaginary substance called black bile were the four humors, or liquids, that kept the body in balance. Too much or too little of any of these would cause disease. They matched up with the elements of fire, water, air, and earth, and with the properties of hot and cold, wet and dry. So if somebody had a disease that was considered to be cold, a physician would describe foods or medicines that had warm properties, or would encourage the body to make more heat.

Galen's ideas stuck around for a very long time. We still speak of getting a "cold," for example, when we get sick and cough up lots of phlegm. Some doctors of his time said that you should feed a cold and starve a fever; Galen preferred to release the heat by draining out one of the "hot" humors, blood.

And so on the basis of Galen's writings, translated and remixed by dozens of writers through the centuries, bloodletting became one of the common-sense treatments for fevers and other diseases.

George Washington may owe his death to too much bloodletting when he consulted doctors about a minor illness. One of today's foremost medical journals, the *Lancet*, owes its name to the trusty bloodletting tool.

THE LONG PLAGUE

Galen treated soldiers during the plague years during a stint in what is now northern Italy. One of his patients was still ailing when he had to sail away, and reported back that he felt better after he came to the town of Tabia and drank some milk. So Galen wrote about the man's symptoms, his treatment, and a detailed description of Tabia so that readers could try to find a similar place (on a hill, near water, and so on) to raise cows that apparently would have the power of curing "the current pestilence" with their milk.

From Galen's descriptions, we have a pretty good idea that the disease was smallpox. It produced a rash all over the body, often with raised pustules, and black diarrhea that indicated intestinal bleeding. (Some historians read this as measles or typhus instead, but the most common interpretation is smallpox.) Galen called it the "great plague" or the "long plague" because it lasted for years and years.

Galen's treatments probably didn't do much to help sufferers of the pestilence. Even with modern medicine, there was never a cure for smallpox. (Not even the milk of Tabia.) The best a doctor could do was isolate the patient, keep him hydrated, and offer medications to manage the symptoms of pain and fever.

A few years into the plague, in C.E. 169, the disease killed Lucius Verus, one of the two co-emperors. The other ruler, Marcus Aurelius, called for Galen and made him court physician. So many people had died at this point that the emperor had to pay foreign mercenaries to defend Rome, often giving them land in payment. Some historians believe this was the beginning of the end for the Roman Empire; millions had died of the plague, and now some of the empire's enemies owned pieces of its land. Finally, in 180, Marcus Aurelius himself died of the pestilence.

Historians now see the Plague of Galen—also called the Antonine plague after Marcus Aurelius Antoninus's full name—as hastening the downfall of Rome. But it could only have helped Galen's fame.

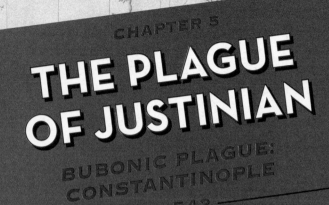

CHAPTER 5

THE PLAGUE OF JUSTINIAN

BUBONIC PLAGUE: CONSTANTINOPLE

C.E. 542

A SHIFT IN WEATHER PATTERNS CAUSES A BOOM IN THE RAT AND FLEA POPULATIONS AND SUDDENLY THE WHOLE OF JUSTINIAN'S EMPIRE IS LAID TO WASTE.

DEATH TOLL: 25 million or more

CAUSED BY: The plague bacterium *Yersinia pestis*

NOTEWORTHY SYMPTOMS: Swollen lymph nodes ("buboes") in groin, armpits, or neck

FATALITY RATE: Unknown, but 60 percent is typical for bubonic plague

THREAT LEVEL TODAY: Low. Plague is rare, and can be treated with antibiotics if caught in time.

NOTABLE FACT: Waves of plague swept over Europe, one after another, for more than 200 years after Justinian's death.

B ubonic plague made its first definite appearance in Western history under the rule of Justinian in the Byzantine Empire. In the shadow of the Hagia Sophia the fleas began to bite, contaminating people's blood with the bacterium *Yersinia pestis*. Shortly thereafter, the people began to die.

"During these times there was a pestilence, by which the whole human race came near to being annihilated," began Procopius, a historian who documented the wars that the emperor Justinian was waging to expand the Byzantine Empire. Procopius traveled and documented battles under the Byzantine general Belisarius, and was present when the plague hit Constantinople in C.E. 542.

The disease struck so heavily that, to the historian, no explanation was possible. It did not prefer a certain season, or country, or people of a given occupation or sex or age. At the height of the outbreak, Procopius wrote, 10,000 people were dying every day. While that number is doubtful only because the Byzantine Empire probably didn't have all that many people, the death toll was certainly enormous.

At first, each family buried their own dead in the usual ways. Soon enough, there were more bodies than places to put them. Families stuffed bodies into other people's tombs. The local government, committed to making sure all the bodies were buried even if they had no family left to do the job, made new cemeteries on every scrap of available land. Soon there were not enough gravediggers to keep up with the enormous task. The city's walls had towers, so that archers could stand at the top to shoot when the city was under attack. Procopius writes that the gravediggers ripped the roofs off these towers, piled bodies inside, and replaced the roofs. When the wind blew, the city was filled with an "evil stench."

WHERE THE PLAGUE CAME FROM

In 542 a global perspective would be impossible—whole continents were unknown to Procopius—but the epidemic included at least the Byzantine Empire, including modern-day Turkey and the ports of the Mediterranean Sea. It spread "as if fearing lest some corner of the earth might escape it." Occasionally a village would be spared, but then the plague would circle back later to take its toll.

Perhaps the plague came, as Procopius said, from Egypt. Today's scientists know that plague infects rodents in many parts of the world, and it has lived in three of these locations longer than others. One is near China, where plague as we know it originated; one runs across the Asian steppe; and the last is in Africa. A few rats could have hopped off a boat from Asia somewhere around Ethiopia, on the eastern coast of Africa, and begun to multiply, like rat pilgrims in a new land.

Whatever the route, somewhere the right kind of rat met the right kind of flea, which was carrying the right kind of bacteria. That bacterium is known today as *Yersinia pestis*, but it has a close relative called *Y. pseudotuberculosis*. The relative lives in the guts of rodents, and relies on one animal ingesting the feces of another. (Don't look so disgusted—if you've ever caught a "stomach flu," that got to you the same way thanks to contaminated food or unwashed hands.)

But *Y. pestis* picked up a couple of tricks that set it free from the fecal-oral path of infection. It can multiply in a rodent or in a person, infecting the bloodstream, and it can survive when eaten as part of a blood meal by a flea. When the rodent dies of plague, the flea hops off, looking for another warm body to feed on—and infect.

THE PLAGUE'S WORLD

Something happened to make the Mediterranean of 542 a great place to be a plague. One possibility is a boom in the rat population. Cold, wet winters often trigger population growth in rodents, and temperature is especially important in plague. The flea likes temperatures in the sixties (Fahrenheit) and one of the plague's favorite ways of spreading, by partially clogging the flea's digestive tract, works best below seventy-five degrees.

It makes sense, then, why the plague spread just a few years after a time when the earth apparently was cooler than usual, as suggested by the growth of tree rings. The reason for the cooling may have been a small comet that crashed into earth, or a volcanic eruption on the other side of the world.

But Procopius had another theory about the disease. After diligently documenting the plague's onset, spread, and symptoms, he wrote his personal take on the cause in another book. Known as *The Secret History* because it wasn't discovered until a millennium later, it describes every type of scandal and debauchery that allegedly went on in the kingdom. There was an obvious reason for the plague, said Procopius: punishment for Justinian's evil ways, including his wholesale slaughter of civilians in the countries he fought.

After devastating the population of the Byzantine Empire and many of its trading partners, the plague burned out. With four months of killing most of the people it met, there probably weren't enough people or rodents to keep passing the bacterium on. The population of susceptible hosts had simply crashed.

The emperor Justinian himself was stricken with plague, and during the weeks while he was on what seemed to be his deathbed, his wife Theodora acted in his stead. After all, not even emperors can hide from disease.

Although Justinian survived, his empire never thrived again. With devastated populations, the empire lost the ground it had gained in decades of expansion through war. Plague had made its mark on Europe, for the first but not the last time.

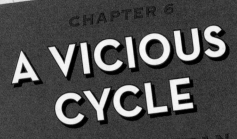

CHAPTER 6

A VICIOUS CYCLE

SMALLPOX: JAPAN
C.E. 735

SINCE JAPAN IS AN ISLAND NATION, EPIDEMICS WERE ONCE RARE—WHICH MEANS EACH TIME THEY ARRIVED THE POPULATION WAS TOTALLY VULNERABLE.

DEATH TOLL: Unknown; possibly 1 million

CAUSED BY: The smallpox virus *Variola major*

NOTEWORTHY SYMPTOMS: Fever and a rash of pustules

FATALITY RATE: An estimated one-third of the population died

THREAT LEVEL TODAY: Gone. Smallpox has been eradicated.

NOTABLE FACT: In an effort to placate the people and the gods, the emperor provided emergency food relief and forgave taxes during plague years.

E pidemics hit Japan hard in its early history because the island nation was so sparsely populated and so isolated from contact with the other countries around it. In other places, like China, a disease like smallpox could simmer in a population, infecting children and leaving adults to boast of their status as survivors. But the disease washed over Japan in devastating waves, killing off swaths of population and then disappearing for a generation at a time.

In C.E. 735, the island nation was ripe for another epidemic. Smallpox had probably visited before, but was long gone. The population had been able to grow a bit in its absence, and maybe people were coming into contact with each other a little more in villages. Roads spread from the biggest towns to the capital in Nara. And in several recent years, the harvests had failed. That meant that farmers and villagers were probably badly nourished when smallpox washed up in Dazaifu's port in modern-day Fukuoka, just 120 miles by boat from Korea.

We don't know exactly how the disease got there, but legend traces it to a Japanese fisherman who became lost at sea and ended up on the Korean peninsula. He became infected but made it home before he died. According to the legend, his return sparked the epidemic.

A NEW THREAT

Smallpox is a virus that spreads like wildfire and has a high mortality rate. At least 20 percent of infected people die, but that's an estimate from populations that are used to seeing smallpox. Numbers are hard to pin down for epidemics so far back in history; however, recent times have seen smallpox mortality as high as 80 percent on islands where the population experiences it for the first time.

The main symptom of smallpox is, of course, the "pocks": red spots that become raised and turn into puffy, white, pus-filled blisters. They develop on the face first, then spread down the chest, arms, and legs. The face and hands get more pockmarks than the rest of the body, and we still don't know why.

Some forms of the disease are even more dangerous: if the pustules run together, forming flat areas instead of individual blisters, the skin can slough off in sheets. In another form, no blisters form at all, or they stay below the skin as pockets of blood. This last form, hemorrhagic smallpox, is almost always fatal.

People probably wondered why such a terrible disease would strike so suddenly. Just as Westerners pinned the blame on God and prayed to saints, the people of the Nara period of Japan looked to their pantheon of gods and ghosts. They found there a vengeful spirit that later evolved into *hōsōgami*, the smallpox god. By the 1800s, this god was said to be afraid of the color red and of dogs, and a shrine to him in the home could help a family to recover from the disease.

In 735, the Council of State issued an order that described the course of the disease and included instructions on how to treat patients. After describing the fever, swellings, and diarrhea that are characteristic of the disease, it recommended wrapping the patient's abdomen and hips tightly in hemp or silk cloth. The patient was to be kept warm and fed a thin gruel made from rice.

Recovery was also to be taken seriously: "For twenty days after the illness passes do not carelessly eat raw fish or fresh fruit or vegetables; do not drink water, take a bath, have sex, or force yourself to do anything, or walk in wind or rain. If you overdo it, a relapse will begin immediately." Another document advises against certain vegetables, and gives recipes for makeup that can hide the smallpox scars. Powdered falcon feathers mixed with lard is one suggestion.

EMERGENCY RELIEF

At first, the government's response was two-pronged: religious and medical. They ordered prayers for the local gods on the island of Kyushu, where the outbreak was killing peasants, and told the governors of nearby areas on the larger island, Honshu, to perform purification rituals to prevent the disease's spread.

At the time, the local Shinto gods were moving over to make room for Buddhist worship, too, and the government hedged its bets: Buddhist priests in the area of the outbreak were to read sutras, or scriptures, too. "The court's heavy reliance on religion may mean that medical remedies were proving ineffective against the killer infection," writes William Farris in *Population, Disease, and Land in Early Japan*. The outbreak continued, and thanks to careful government records from the time, which Farris pieces together, we can see just how bad it was.

The emperor was able to make special grants of rice available in bad times, as a form of emergency relief when harvests failed. In 735, he issued grain for a new reason—to the victims of the epidemic. The government of Kyushu made a special request that the island population's tax be forgiven for that year, because "the whole populace is bedridden." The request was granted.

The emperor offered amnesty for the entire country after that, but the disease continued to spread. The next year, grain and medicine were to be sent to all monks, nuns, and commoners who were afflicted. Soon it affected the aristocracy, too.

A diplomatic mission from the Japanese capital crossed through plague-worn areas on their way to Korea. They never made it to their destination. The group's leader died and was buried on Tsushima Island, the halfway point, and the survivors straggled back, spreading smallpox to new areas and to the ruling classes. The powerful Fujiwara clan was headed by four brothers, and all four caught smallpox and died.

The emperor was also ready to shake things up himself. "Bad omens are still to be seen," he wrote. "I fear the responsibility is all mine." Farris suggests that the emperor channeled his guilt into support of the newish religion of Buddhism. He ordered Buddhist temples to be built all over the country, and built a giant bronze and gold Buddha statue and a museum of medicinal herbs. The disease stayed away, but not for long. It returned in 763, then 790, and sporadically for centuries.

The country was caught in a vicious cycle: its small, sparse population meant that disease could never settle in and give people an opportunity to become immune. As soon as the population recovered from each outbreak, a new one would strike, reducing the population yet again. Finally, around the year 1000, Japan's population was finally able to grow—around the same time that smallpox became a tragic but common childhood disease.

CHAPTER 7

MESSAGE FROM A SACRED MOUNTAIN

SMALLPOX: CHINA

c. 1000

IN THIS CHINESE EPIDEMIC, ONE OFFICIAL IS FED UP WITH SMALLPOX—AND LEARNS THE SECRET OF PREVENTING EPIDEMICS EVER AFTERWARD.

DEATH TOLL: Unknown

CAUSED BY: The smallpox virus *Variola major*

NOTEWORTHY SYMPTOMS: Fever and a rash of pustules

FATALITY RATE: Unknown; 20 percent in later epidemics

THREAT LEVEL TODAY: Gone. Smallpox has been eradicated through worldwide vaccination.

NOTABLE FACT: This epidemic's legacy was an early form of immunization practiced in many parts of the world.

Around the turn of the first millennium, an epidemic of small-pox broke out in Song Dynasty China. The disease wasn't new to China, and was probably well on its way to being a "childhood disease"—one that only struck children because adults had all lived through previous epidemics.

After this time, though, things would be different. A high-ranking official named Wang Dan had lost children to the disease during the previous epidemic. He now had another son, and didn't want to lose him too. Wang Dan called for physicians and priests from all over the newly unified nation to come and share their advice.

One of the guests was a Taoist nun who lived in one of the temples on Mount Emei. She showed Wang Dan how to inoculate a person against smallpox, grinding up the scabs from a mild case of the disease and puffing them up the person's nose. She was an incarnation of the goddess of mercy, people said, come to save the lives of children. While inoculation is certainly an ancient practice, we don't really know when or where it started. The more picturesque details may just be artistic license. The Song Dynasty was in power around C.E. 1000, but the earliest surviving document that describes the legend was written in 1695. By then, physician Zhang Lu wrote, the technique was widespread.

The Chinese method was a little different from the vaccines that eventually caught on in Europe. In China, practitioners made sure that people gaining protection would get it the same way they would naturally: by inhaling it. The people who performed the inoculations would take the scabs from smallpox patients, grind them into powder, and wear the vial of powder next to their skin for a few weeks, letting heat and time kill off some of the virus. When the time came to inoculate, the practitioner would put some of the powdered scabs into a long metal pipe and gently blow the disease up the person's nose.

A SMART STRATEGY

Inoculation rarely caused cases of full-blown smallpox. Aging the scabs probably helped. Another part of the strategy was to only take smallpox scabs from people who had mild cases of the disease. We know today that there is actually more than one type of smallpox: *Variola major* causes the infamous type, the one that kills around 25 percent of the people who contract it. But *Variola minor* has a fatality rate of 3 percent or less. Cultures that practiced inoculation typically used the mildest strains they could find—these may have been *V. minor*, or at least a weak *V. major*. It also probably helped to use the pustules triggered by somebody else's inoculation than to take them from a sufferer in the throes of the full-blown disease.

China was not the only place where inoculation was traditional. There is evidence of some form of inoculation in India, the Middle East, and Africa. For example, Cotton Mather, a Puritan in Massachusetts, asked his slave Onesimus if he had ever had smallpox. "Yes and no," the man said, showing a scar on his arm. Back home, he said, children got smallpox in an operation and were then protected for life. A few years later, Mather read about the same operation in a British medical journal; a doctor from Constantinople wrote that the practice was common there.

Onesimus came from western Africa, around present-day Burkina Faso. Some form of inoculation—usually putting smallpox pus into a cut on the healthy person's arm—was also practiced in eastern parts of Africa, and in the Ottoman Empire (modern-day Turkey).

Europe was among the last places to take up inoculation. Physicians there thought that smallpox pustules were bad humors created in the body, rising to the surface. What good would it do to introduce more of a bad humor? In China, the idea caught on quicker because doctors there had a different idea of where disease comes from. All children are born with a poison inside them, the theory went. Triggering a mild case of smallpox would use up some of that poison, so the child would not get sick in the future.

EUROPE CATCHES ON

Finally, Lady Mary Wortley Montagu made inoculation fashionable. She was a social climber with beauty, wit, money, and royal friends—but one day smallpox removed beauty from the equation. She survived a bout of the disease, badly scarred, and thankful that her infant son hadn't caught it from her.

On a trip to the Ottoman Empire with her ambassador husband, Lady Mary learned about inoculation. She wrote to a friend about the old women who would come around in the spring with a nutshell full of "the best sort" of smallpox pus, and insert some in your veins. Children have a few days of fever and a few pustules that don't leave scars.

Lady Mary had the procedure done on her son, and back in England she convinced Princess Caroline to inoculate the royal grandchildren. Physicians argued against the idea at first, saying that something practiced by women in a supposedly less civilized country couldn't possibly be better than European medicine.

They couldn't deny the results, though: inoculation carried a 1 percent fatality rate, while natural smallpox killed 20 percent of patients. In an attempt to make inoculation fit with their understanding of the body, physicians soon turned inoculation into a weeks-long process that required bloodletting and special diets.

Physician Edward Jenner was looking to streamline this process when he learned about a farmer who had inoculated his family with the cow version of smallpox. Jenner experimented on a local boy, and called the successful result his *vaccine*, from the Latin word for cow.

Skeptics of the day made fun of the vaccine, suggesting that it would give people horns and other cow-like qualities. But using a virus that was milder and different from smallpox was a smart idea—one worthy of the goddess of mercy herself.

CHAPTER 8

SAINT ANTHONY'S FIRE

ERGOTISM: FRANCE
1095

UNLUCKY PEASANTS COULD LOSE THEIR LIMBS TO ERGOT POISONING, HALLUCINATING ALL THE WHILE—GIVING NEW MEANING TO THE PHRASE "WATCH WHAT YOU EAT."

DEATH TOLL: Unknown; one epidemic in C.E. 944 killed 40,000 people

CAUSED BY: A fungus that grows on grain, *Claviceps purpurea*

NOTEWORTHY SYMPTOMS: Burning pain, hallucinations, gangrene

FATALITY RATE: Estimated at 40 percent

THREAT LEVEL TODAY: Low, now that we know that grain with this fungus is unfit for consumption.

NOTABLE FACT: The hallucinations came from a natural chemical in the ergot that works in the brain like a chemical we know today: LSD.

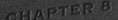

For centuries, it wasn't a big deal that some of the rye would occasionally be black at harvest time. That's just how rye sometimes was. Among the grains clustered at the top of each stalk, the black ones would be extra long, sometimes three times as long as the regular grain. Maybe some people tried to pick them out before grinding the rye into flour; others, especially in times of famine, would eat them anyway. One German word for the black grains was *Hungerkorn*.

Nobody made the connection, at first, to a horrific malady that would strike whole villages at a time. It caused a burning pain, especially in the arms and legs. Some people experienced convulsions and would lie in bed twitching, necks twisted in agony. Others would find that their fiery limbs would turn black and cease to ache; gangrene took over and the limb would, eventually, fall off. Pregnant women would go into labor, whether or not their doomed babies were ready to be born.

The disease struck so suddenly and horribly that to some it seemed like a divine or demonic curse. *Ignis sacer* was one name for it: holy fire.

They didn't realize that the symptoms all came from the *Hungerkorn*, and that the black grains were created by a fungus now called *Claviceps purpurea*. It consumes the grain as it grows, and in the winter the black grains form tiny mushroom-like structures to disperse spores. While many grains are susceptible to ergot fungus, rye—eaten largely by the poor—was its most common host in medieval Europe. The fungus grows best in cool, wet weather, so wet years became years of widespread holy fire. In 1095, with no cause or cure in sight, some religious people opened a hospital dedicated to treating the disorder. They would eventually run an international network of more than 300 hospitals.

THE HOSPITAL BROTHERS OF SAINT ANTHONY

The brothers took their name from Saint Anthony. This saint, the story goes, was one of the first religious hermits. A bishop who had met him wrote down his life story: Anthony sold his possessions to benefit the poor and lived alone in the desert. There, the devil whispered to him about the wealth and family he had left behind, about good food, about sex. (Especially about sex.) The devil even appeared to Saint Anthony in the form of a woman, but with the Lord's strength, the biographer wrote, the saint rejected all of the devil's temptations. Over time, the hallucinations of ergotism came to be linked to the visions Saint Anthony had in the desert.

Documents from one German hospital describe how the pilgrims were received. First, three surgeons would decide whether the new person was actually suffering from the holy fire, comparing the symptoms with those of the other patients. The patient could stay for a lifetime if he had the gangrenous form of the disease and required amputation. If he only had the milder form, with convulsions and hallucinations, he could stay nine days and then had to leave to make room for the next pilgrim.

The patient would confess his sins and attend the day's church services, and then take vows of chastity and prayer. Health of the body and spirit were connected, the monks believed. Once the patient was committed to this religious cure, he could take his first sip of the famous Antonite wine.

PUTTING OUT THE FIRE

We don't know what was in the wines or herbal ointments that the Antonites used, but there are some clues. Medieval medical texts sometimes include nightshades, like mandrake or henbane, in the treatment of holy fire; one salve calls for crushing the seeds of the poppy in vinegar. The result would be an opium ointment that might be able to relieve pain.

Another clue comes from a wooden altarpiece at one of the St. Anthony churches. It was painted by Matthias Grünewald, who had lived with the Antonites and may have suffered from holy fire himself. In one panel, two saints sit with plants growing near their feet. The plants appear to be fourteen local species exactingly rendered, perhaps a hint for identifying the ingredients needed in the medicines.

However, the monks' real secret may have had nothing to do with the medicines. Since the Antonites supplied food for the patients, and the patients may have traveled many miles from their home, a big advantage of staying with the Antonites may just have been a separate food supply. As long as the hospital's fields didn't use the black grain, the food there would have been safe.

Some modern historians believe the wines and ointments would have included pain relievers and ingredients that could counteract the blood vessel constriction that caused the burning and gangrene. On the other hand, Galen's theories of balancing humors were still in force. A disease characterized by burning would have been treated with foods and medicines that were categorized as cold. The fruit of the mandrake plant was one of these. But that fruit, a nightshade, was hallucinogenic.

And so a person under the care of the monks might be experiencing hallucinations from both the medication and the disease. This may be why Saint Anthony's temptations evolved over the years, from the devil whispering in the desert to torturous scenes of suffering creatures. Grünewald's altarpiece opposite the panel with the plants shows a man fending off attacks from a bird-headed creature, and others with disembodied limbs and objects bearing faces. A burned building is in the background; a pregnant woman is naked and covered in sores, her neck contorted, her feet replaced with duck's feet. Other artists continued in this theme, from Hieronymus Bosch's contorted demons to Salvador Dali's scene in which the saint fends off a parade of stilt-legged elephants.

Later, scientists figured out that ergot was the cause of Saint Anthony's fire. In 1938, a chemist investigating ergot made a synthetic drug that mimicked some of its properties. This was the famous LSD. Hippies flocked to it for the psychedelic effects, leaving ergotism's agonizing symptoms—the burning and the gangrene— to the dustbin of history.

CHAPTER 9

A DOOMED CRUSADE

SCURVY: EGYPT
1249

CRUSADING KNIGHTS KNEW THEIR TRIP WOULD BE DANGEROUS, BUT THEY PROBABLY WEREN'T EXPECTING THEIR BODIES TO LITERALLY FALL APART. IF ONLY THEY'D KNOWN ABOUT VITAMINS!

DEATH TOLL: Unknown

CAUSED BY: Lack of vitamin C in the diet

NOTEWORTHY SYMPTOMS: Fatigue, bruises and bleeding from the skin, swollen legs and gums

FATALITY RATE: 100 percent if untreated

THREAT LEVEL TODAY: Low

NOTABLE FACT: Weakness due to rampant disease among the Crusaders may be partly to blame for the French king being captured and held for ransom.

War is unhealthy in many ways. Violent injuries, poor living conditions, and lack of healthy food set the stage for immense suffering even aside from tragic battlefield deaths. But for the French soldiers in the Seventh Crusade, one cause stood out above the others: clearly they could blame eels.

Eels, after all, eat the dead. At least that's what Jean de Joinville believed. He documented the crusade, in which King Louis IX of France intended to take Jerusalem back from Muslim control. To get to that city, the king figured he needed to capture some prime territory in Egypt. And that's where the Crusaders ran into trouble.

They captured an Egyptian port called Damietta, then moved up the Nile to attack Al Mansurah. When that went disastrously wrong, they retreated to their camp on the river bank. And there, instead of the Crusaders seizing a city, they themselves were seized.

The enemy set up ships between their camp and Damietta to cut off supplies. The Crusaders could not send for the salt beef and salt pork they had left in Damietta, but it didn't matter anyway. The season was Lent, and by religious law they could not eat meat most days of the week, only fish. And fish proved hard to come by, so they went with the next best thing: eels.

The bodies from the last battle were still floating in the river, but the Nile had flooded so that the water was even with the bridge near the Crusaders' camp. So the bodies could not float past the bridge, and stayed there until the king hired local help to bury the Christians and throw the rest over the bridge downstream.

In the meantime, Jean de Joinville figured the eels must have been eating the bodies, and so when the people ate the eels, they caught some contagion of death. The Crusaders had begun to feel fatigued, and soon their legs were covered in black marks and bruises, some tiny like dots and some massive, swollen, and bleeding. Their gums also swelled. "None escaped this sickness save through the jaws of death," he wrote. He didn't have a name for this disease, but it was scurvy.

The king developed the disease, as did huge numbers of the men, making them too weak to fight. If the crusade was not doomed from the beginning, it surely was now.

Joinville was wounded in battle and had a fever in addition to the scurvy. Among the injured, underfed population, multiple diseases were probably routine. Scurvy is bad, but scurvy plus typhus or dysentery would be worse. Joinville had a priest say a mass for him when he thought he was on his deathbed. The priest, also sick, collapsed in the middle of a song. Joinville leaped out of bed to hold the priest tight and tell him he must finish the mass. The priest did, and perished. Joinville lived.

Later, Joinville writes that barbers (who wielded knives for any part of the body in that day, not just the hair) helped the sufferers by cutting away the swollen gum tissue from their teeth so they would be able to eat. "A most piteous thing it was," he wrote, "to hear through the camp the screams of the people from whom they were cutting the dead flesh, for they screamed just like women labouring with child."

VITAMIN C

Scurvy comes not from eels, of course, but from a lack of vitamin C. This tiny molecule, found in many fruits and vegetables (especially citrus fruit), is necessary for the body to make collagen.

Ropes of protein called collagen are the main ingredients in the connective tissues that hold the human body together. There is collagen in our gums, in our skin, and in bones and muscle. It's strong and stretchy, and without it we begin to fall apart. This is what happens in scurvy. Normally collagen is built, and constantly rebuilt, by enzymes that require iron and vitamin C to keep them functional. Without healthy collagen, tissues soften and blood leaks out.

We need about 60 milligrams of vitamin C every day, easy to get from any of a variety of fresh fruits or vegetables. The body can store anywhere between 900 and 1,500 milligrams. If you quit eating foods with vitamin C, you would stay healthy for two or three months, thanks to the stored vitamin.

But when body levels drop below about 500 milligrams, the symptoms of scurvy start to show up. One of the first signs is fatigue. Then come muscle pain and tiny blood-filled spots on the limbs. A small dose of the vitamin, at this point, might not be enough to bring the body's vitamin C levels back to normal. If you have a few oranges handy, this would be a good time to start eating them.

SCURVY TODAY

Scurvy occasionally pops up today amid famines or natural disasters. Otherwise it is so rare that individual cases of it, in high-income nations, are published as medical oddities.

One of these was a woman in Denmark, described in the *Journal of Clinical Medicine Research* in 2012, who had weight-loss surgery. This procedure works by making it harder for the body to absorb calories from food, but it can also mean that the body absorbs fewer vitamins and minerals. Patients are supposed to make sure to take vitamins and to eat a healthy diet, but the woman was so enthusiastic about her weight loss that she ate next to nothing for months on end. By the time she showed up at the hospital, she was in a state probably not too different from that of the Crusaders (minus the typhoid and dysentery). Her skin was covered in bruises and huge pockets of blood; she lost an enormous amount of blood every day just through her skin.

The doctors thought at first that she had a life-threatening infection, possibly coming from wounds on her legs. Her organs were shutting down—including her brain, lungs, heart, and kidneys. The medical team put her onto a ventilator to help her breathe, and hooked her up to a dialysis machine to take over for her failing kidneys. And then somebody thought to test her for scurvy. She didn't have an infection, after all. To the IV lines entering her veins, they began adding large doses of vitamin C. Just two days later, her skin began to recover. Within a few weeks, her lungs and kidneys were again working on their own. Some of the Crusaders recovered, too, but not until after battles had been lost and their king captured.

CHAPTER 10

THE KNIGHTS OF LAZARUS

LEPROSY (HANSEN'S DISEASE): EUROPE

1200s

LEPROSY IS NOT VERY CONTAGIOUS, WE KNOW TODAY, AND MOST PEOPLE ARE IMMUNE TO IT. SO WHY DID EUROPEANS SUDDENLY BUILD SO MANY LEPER COLONIES? AND HOW DID IT DISAPPEAR JUST AS SUDDENLY?

DEATH TOLL: Up to 20 percent of the population in some areas

CAUSED BY: The bacterium *Mycobacterium leprae*

NOTEWORTHY SYMPTOMS: Rough, thickened skin; loss of fingers and toes

FATALITY RATE: Hansen's disease is not fatal by itself, but people with the disease are at increased risk of contracting (and dying from) other infections

THREAT LEVEL TODAY: Low. The disease still exists in some countries, but can be treated with antibiotics.

NOTABLE FACT: Many leprosaria (leper colonies) were run as democracies, with participation open to both men and women.

So many warriors came down with leprosy during the Crusades that they had their own fighting order. Next to the Knights Templar, the Knights Hospitaller, and the Equestrian Order of the Holy Sepulchre was the Order of Saint Lazarus.

The Knights Templar, for example, had a rule that if one of their members contracted the disease, he had the choice of either living in isolation or joining the Knights of Lazarus. The Templars would pay for his food and expenses, but he would fight with the Lazarites in battle, wearing their symbol, the green cross.

The group began with a leprosarium just outside the wall of Jerusalem. At first, the monks' mission was simply to care for the sick there. Even during and after the Crusades, it seems that members could join to care for the people who lived at this leprosarium and, later, others that the group founded. Some were able to fight, but when they became too weak they could return to the leprosarium, where their stronger brothers would care for them.

Leprosy, which we know today as Hansen's disease, is rare and does not spread easily. But historical records show that it was probably common in the Middle East then. Jerusalem had even had a "leper king" who contracted the disease in childhood but still led armies in battle and ruled the country from age thirteen until his death at twenty-four.

Around the same time, leprosy became common in Europe. Perhaps Crusaders brought it back when they returned. By 1240, leprosaria like the one at Jerusalem dotted the European continent. Every major city had at least one. In total, there may have been thousands.

A PARADOX

The image of leprosy as a highly contagious disease sweeping across a continent just doesn't fit with what we know about it today. Hansen's disease—historically lumped together with other skin conditions under the name "leprosy"—is not very contagious. It may spread from person to person through nasal droplets, for example from a sneeze. But not everybody on the receiving end of a sneeze will develop symptoms. People with Hansen's disease often have roommates or family members who take years to get sick, if they even get sick at all. Ninety-five percent of people can't even catch the disease.

But we're not looking at a case of mistaken identity; DNA analysis in graveyards shows that the people who died in leprosaria were infected with the same bacterium that Dr. Gerhard Henrik Armauer Hansen found in 1873 when he peered down his microscope at a snippet of skin from a leprosy patient.

Hansen's disease is an infection by a very odd bacterium called *Mycobacterium leprae*. It grows slowly, and takes different forms depending on how the person's body fights the disease. The less severe form causes numbness that can lead to infected injuries in the hands and feet; people with this form can end up losing their fingers and toes. The more severe form swells and thickens earlobes, facial skin, and other body parts. People with this form can suffocate if the disease blocks their nose and throat, or go blind if it infects their eyes.

THE DECLINE AND FALL OF LEPROSY

In medieval Europe, plenty of diseases were more contagious and more dangerous than leprosy. So why was it the one disease that could make a person into an outcast?

Part of the answer may lie in a misunderstanding of a passage from the Old Testament. In Leviticus, the same book that declares pork to be always unclean and people who have had sex to be unclean until evening, a skin condition called *tzaraath* makes people so unclean they must live outside the camp or the city until it clears up.

While later this was translated as *leprae*, it isn't strictly leprosy. A person can recover from *tzaraath*, whereas Hansen's disease is incurable. The book also includes descriptions of *tzaraath* on clothing and houses, which probably referred to something like a mold or mildew.

Centuries later, religious people of Europe struggled with understanding leprosy. On the one hand, Jesus had cured lepers. Suffering led to holiness, according to an idea of the time, so perhaps people with the disease are blessed. On the other hand, leprosy was sometimes seen as a punishment for sins. And so the leprosaria of Europe were part charity, where the faithful could minister to the sick; part religious order, where people with leprosy prayed and tried to live holy lives; and part prison, where people could end up if a council (which may not have included any doctors) ruled that they were lepers.

And yet, the population of people with leprosy declined suddenly and sharply in the 1300s. One factor may have been the "leper massacre" of 1321. The leprosaria of the Knights of Lazarus governed themselves democratically, and as the organization grew it amassed wealth and power. This threatened King Philip V of France. He accused the organization of conspiring to poison all the non-lepers in Europe. He probably invented the idea as a political move to let him dissolve the organization and take their land, but people took matters into their own hands and killed lepers en masse. The king retracted his accusation, but it was too late.

This can't be the only explanation, though. Leprosarium graveyards have been found in Denmark, and the burials show that leprosy—actual Hansen's disease—was common in the 1200s but disappeared after 1400 or so. Why?

One theory is that tuberculosis began to spread throughout Europe. Tuberculosis is closely related to leprosy, enough that it may have been able to serve as a natural vaccine. On the other hand, maybe the leprosaria themselves deserve the credit: isolating people with the disease may have helped to halt its spread. Or, since not everybody is susceptible, people with the genes to resist leprosy may have come to take over the population, leaving few people available to pass on the bacterium.

Even today, Hansen's disease is something of a mystery to scientists, who are still learning about who contracts it and why it makes the body respond the way it does. There is still one more possibility that doesn't rely on changes in people's genetics: maybe the lepers and their caretakers were wiped out by another epidemic. The timing is right: in the middle of the 1300s, a new disease marched up the continent. It was called the Black Death.

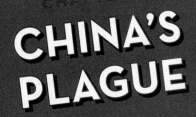

CHINA'S PLAGUE

THE "BLACK DEATH" THAT DEVASTATED EUROPE STARTED FIRST IN CHINA, AND PROBABLY RODE ACROSS THE STEPPE ON HORSEBACK.

DEATH TOLL: Unknown, but very large

CAUSED BY: The bacterium *Yersinia pestis*

NOTEWORTHY SYMPTOMS: Swollen lymph nodes ("buboes") in groin, armpits, or neck

FATALITY RATE: Unknown, but 60 percent is typical for bubonic plague

THREAT LEVEL TODAY: Low. Plague is rare, and can be treated with antibiotics if caught in time.

NOTABLE FACT: Legends say that in China and India just before the plague, the earth shook and frogs and serpents rained down.

I t began, perhaps, with a tarbagan.

A tarbagan is a type of marmot, a creature that looks like a groundhog and is about the size of a rabbit, with soft fur and tasty meat. Tarbagans live like prairie dogs in burrows in central Asia, roughly where Mongolia is today, and they are known to be susceptible to bubonic plague.

The people who hunt tarbagans today have a taboo on shooting a rodent that is staggering or moving slowly. Carefully avoiding sick animals may be what kept plague contained in the first place. But one day, it seems, somebody killed the wrong tarbagan, and sparked a pandemic.

The Plague of Justinian was an earlier branch from this same ancestral ground. In 2011, an international team of researchers reported that they constructed plague's family tree by comparing many modern samples of the bacterium that causes it, *Yersinia pestis*. The germ is now found worldwide, not just across Asia and Europe but also entrenched in Africa, Madagascar, and the southwestern United States.

If two samples were similar, the researchers' computer programs put them together on the family tree, like brothers. A slightly more different sample would be on a nearby branch, like a cousin, and so on until they reached the branches of the family that were the least related to each other. Those were only linked by ancestors from very long ago.

Samples from China were on every branch, including the oldest ones. Their conclusion, which they published in *Nature Genetics*: "Our observations thus suggest that *Yersinia pestis* evolved in China and spread to other areas again and again."

That means that if Procopius had seen Justinian's plague coming from Egypt, that was just a way station on a much longer journey it had taken from central Asia. Nearly a thousand years later, in the 1300s, the plague seems to have set off from its home once again.

ON THE ROAD

Unlike earlier outbreaks, this time the plague had an open road stretching out before it. Genghis Khan, 150 years before, had conquered vast swaths of the continent. He set up a long-distance messenger service across the steppe, sort of a pony express that nobody would dare attack. Routes became available for armies and commercial caravans, whose bustling businesses brought Arabian horses to China and Chinese silk to the Middle East. Marco Polo traveled these routes; so did a French ambassador who discovered, in the Mongol capital Karakorum, that a woman he met had been kidnapped years before from a village near his own hometown.

The plague germ had an advantage that helped it to travel long distances: somebody who contracted plague could hop on a horse and be hundreds of miles away before coming down with symptoms. By that point the person would most likely be in a camp, where there were plenty of rats to carry on the next plague-filled flea. Eventually, that flea could infect another person.

Only in recent years have scientists begun to appreciate the plague bacterium's tricks. It evolved from a gut microbe that had a simple tactic: grow in a rodent's intestines, get pooped out, contaminate some food, get eaten, and begin the cycle again. (Its distant relative *Yersinia pseudotuberculosis* still works that way.) But *Y. pestis* found its way into the bloodstream, where it could be picked up by a flea. There, it needs to survive in the flea's gut before it can be injected into the next rodent.

Y. pestis doesn't depend on just one species of rat, or just one species of flea. Besides the tarbagan and the black rat, plague can also be carried by prairie dogs, ground squirrels, gerbils, and many other rodents. And it can jump from animal to animal via 80 species of fleas associated with 200 different kinds of rodents.

In some, like the rat flea *Xenopsylla cheopis*, the plague bacterium forms a sticky clot in the flea's gut, causing it to spit out plague-contaminated blood whenever it bites a new victim. In others, like the human flea *Pulex irritans*, plague's only route is to cling for dear life to the flea's bloody mouthparts, and hope it bites another person soon. Scientists argue over which route is more efficient, but both work.

When *Y. pestis* finally gets into a person's bloodstream, it deploys many chemical weapons. For example, it turns off a protein that helps it survive in the flea's gut, and turns on another that helps it avoid the human (or rodent) immune system.

White blood cells called macrophages normally eat invading bacteria, and take them to lymph nodes. *Y. pestis* can avoid being eaten, or it can allow itself to be eaten and prevent the macrophage from digesting and killing it. So when the white blood cell arrives at a lymph node—normally in the groin, if it came from a flea bite on the foot or leg—*Y. pestis* is alive and well. It multiplies there, turning the lymph node into a painful lump called a bubo that can swell as large as an egg or even a baseball. At the same time, it also takes over other organs, including the liver and spleen, turning them into factories for making more *Y. pestis*.

And amazingly, this whole time it manages to silence the cells it kills, preventing them from alerting the rest of the immune system. Until the germs complete their takeover, the person—or rat—has no idea they are sick. But in the end, from the germ's point of view, the host must die. A flea will stay for life on a warm, hairy body. When that animal dies and the body goes cold, the flea jumps off, with plague-infected gut or mouthparts, to find its next meal.

LEAVING FOOTPRINTS

We don't have gripping narrative accounts of the plague in China the way we do for the branch that hit Europe. William McNeill, when writing his influential book *Plagues and Peoples*, asked a Chinese-speaking colleague, Joseph Cha, to find evidence of epidemics in ancient China. The results show the footprints of a deadly plague, although we can't be sure that *Yersinia pestis* was the culprit in each case. For example, after a series of smaller epidemics in modern-day Hubei, a massive epidemic beginning in 1331 killed

90 percent of the population. Smaller epidemics followed in Fujian and Shandong in 1345 and 1346.

At the same time, the plague must have also been creeping westward from its starting point. A small Christian community just west of China, near Lake Issyk-Kul, has just a handful of graves for each year—except 1339, when there are over 100. One inscription, still readable, says: "This is the grave of Kutluk. He died of plague with his wife Mangu-kelka."

The plague reached Caffa (now Feodosia) in Crimea in 1347, and from there raged through Europe. Meanwhile it was still on the march in China: a 1351 epidemic killed half the army in the Huai Valley. In 1353, two-thirds of the population of Shanxi died. In 1354, disease claimed over 60 percent of the people of Hebei. In total, from 1200 until the Ming Dynasty replaced Mongol rule, the population of the area we now know as China was cut in half, from 123 million to just 65 million. War and famine accounted for some of the deaths, but plague must have taken a huge toll.

The Muslim scholar Ibn al-Wardi wrote a brief history of the disease when it arrived in the Middle East in 1348. It had been sweeping Asia for fifteen years, from what he had heard. "China could not be preserved from it," he wrote; the plague "afflicted India," "attacked Persia," and "gnawed" at the Crimea. Upon reaching Aleppo, his home in what is now Syria, he wrote that it brought entire families to their graves in two or three nights.

The plague killed Ibn al-Wardi himself the following year. By then, it was already in England, having clawed its way upward through Europe. The Black Death was not done yet.

CHAPTER 12

THE BLACK DEATH

BUBONIC PLAGUE: EUROPE
1348

THE MOST INFAMOUS OF ALL PLAGUES, AND PERHAPS THE MOST DEADLY, THE BLACK DEATH REACHED EVERY CORNER OF EUROPE, SLAUGHTERING MANY AND SPARING FEW.

DEATH TOLL: Estimated at one-third of the population of Europe, perhaps 25 million

CAUSED BY: The bacterium *Yersinia pestis*

NOTEWORTHY SYMPTOMS: Swollen lymph nodes ("buboes") in groin, armpits, or neck

FATALITY RATE: Unknown, but 60 percent is typical for bubonic plague

THREAT LEVEL TODAY: Low. Plague is rare, and can be treated with antibiotics if caught in time.

NOTABLE FACT: At the time, there was no medicine effective against the plague, but sweet-smelling scents were thought to be protective.

Death was not new to the people of medieval Europe. Other diseases made the rounds regularly; one in four infants died before their first birthday. But the plague was terror like they had never seen before.

Fear is a survival strategy. It helps us to protect ourselves. But it also motivates terrible treatment of our fellow humans. In plagues, people flee when they see the disease approaching. It's common to abandon a home, a town—temporarily, people tell themselves—and in the Black Death the fear was so great that people gave up on their loved ones.

"Father abandoned child, wife husband, one brother another," writes a chronicler in Siena, Italy, "for this illness seemed to strike through breath and sight. And so they died." Gravediggers and priests were in short supply, so funerals often didn't happen, he writes. Instead, "all were thrown in those ditches and covered with earth. And as soon as those ditches were filled, more were dug. I, Agnolo di Tura, called the Fat, buried my five children with my own hands, and so did many others likewise."

Europeans gave the plague names like the Great Mortality. "Black Death" was a name that came later, from historians looking back. Archaeologists have found *Yersinia pestis* DNA in mass graves from the time, confirming that this pandemic was indeed the work of the germ that causes bubonic plague. (The same germ, when spread by coughing, creates the faster-killing "pneumonic" plague. Both were probably at work in the Black Death.)

The plague may have entered Europe through the Crimean port of Caffa, now called Feodosia. In 1347 it belonged to the Genoese, and was surrounded—on the land side, anyway—by attacking Mongols. In one account, the Mongols began to die of the plague, and took advantage of the situation by catapulting corpses over the city walls. In another version, the Mongols decided the plague was a sign from God that their religion was the wrong one, so they decided to convert to Christianity. Upon entering the city, they found the Christian population had been devastated just like theirs.

RELIGION AND SCAPEGOATS

Ships full of plague sufferers sailed for Italy. One of these tried to land at Messina, in Sicily, with "sickness clinging to their very bones." The locals turned them away, but it was too late—some person, or some rat, had sparked an epidemic in the town. The people of Messina went to nearby Catania for help. At first the Catanians treated them in their hospitals, but when plague began to spread there too, they stopped accepting newcomers.

Messina was doomed. Catania's archbishop attempted to help by bringing some specially blessed holy water, but according to legend he arrived to find the city full of demons in the shape of dogs. The people of Messina then went to another town to borrow another holy relic, but the horse carrying it refused to enter the doomed city.

In Milan, three households were found to have plague, and the people walled up those houses and left the inhabitants for dead. In Pistoia, city officials decreed that residents would not be allowed to re-enter the city if they had traveled to an area with plague. That decree came along with another saying that funeral bells would no longer be rung (presumably they were already ringing nonstop). A later update banned funeral candles, since the city was running out of wax.

In Germany, there was already a thriving cult of "flagellants," people who whipped themselves in public ceremonies as a penance for the community. They marched from town to town, putting on three of these shows per day. Once the plague arrived, the flagellants announced that a letter had been hand-delivered from God by an angel, stating that the people of Europe were sinners and needed to whip themselves more.

But the most harmful religious fear was the idea that plague came from a conspiracy to poison water supplies. The fact that plague killed people of all religions didn't stop town officials from arresting and torturing Jews. In 1348, a man who had been "put to torture a little" confessed to picking up a packet of poison on a business trip to Venice and sprinkling it in the water supply of every town he passed on the way home. In the areas now known as southern France, Spain, Switzerland, and Germany, town after town rounded up the local Jewish populations for horrific punishments. Often, they were burned to death.

MEDICINE WAS USELESS

The pope, then headquartered at Avignon in France, wrote orders condemning the flagellants' ceremonies and the persecution of Jews. But he did so from the comfort of the papal bedroom, where, per doctor's orders, he refused visitors and sat between two fires.

Physicians of the time still based their practice on Galen's ancient texts about the four humors, by then copied umpteen times in Latin. The body needed to have its humors (blood, phlegm, black bile, yellow bile) in the proper balance to avoid sickness.

Manipulating your food or environment, according to this idea, could rebalance your humors. The ancient Greeks, probably connecting warm swampy places with sickness like malaria, declared that "hot" and "wet" properties could make a person sick. Blood is also considered to be hot and wet, so removing a few pints of blood from a plague sufferer sounded like a good idea. Bloodletting was a treatment for almost any illness from Hippocrates's time up until the era of germ theory in the nineteenth century.

So the pope's fires were likely meant to dry the air. Plague sufferers were also advised to eat their meat roasted (dry) rather than boiled (wet).

Doctors of the time recommended burning strong-smelling herbs in the fire, like juniper or rosemary, since disease was also linked with tainted air. In medieval cities, smells of rotting garbage and animal waste would have been normal. In a time of pestilence, with dead bodies littering the streets, the smell must have been unbearable. Wealthy patients could have a "smelling apple" made out of a paste of sandalwood, camphor, pepper, and roses to hold up to their noses when they left the house.

The king of France wanted a scientific answer to the question on everybody's mind: Why did this plague come to destroy us? The Medical Faculty of Paris matter-of-factly looked to the stars. Saturn, Mars, and Jupiter had come together in the constellation of Aquarius, they said, which was a hot, wet sign. Aristotle had written that "mortality of races and the depopulation of kingdoms" happen when Saturn and Jupiter get together, and adding Mars to the mix makes matters worse. Jupiter draws up evil vapors from the earth, and Mars ignites them. This explains the recent storms and earthquakes, they said. The plague had only just arrived, but the stars were clear about the city's prognosis. The report stated, simply, "we fear that we are in for an epidemic."

CHAPTER 13

THE SWEATING SICKNESS

UNKNOWN DISEASE: ENGLAND
1485

Sweating was the least of your worries if you were struck with this illness. It killed so quickly you barely had time for a fever before you died.

DEATH TOLL: 15,000 in six weeks

CAUSED BY: Unknown; perhaps a virus of the genus *Hantavirus*

NOTEWORTHY SYMPTOMS: Fever causing extreme sweating; death within hours

FATALITY RATE: 50 percent or more

THREAT LEVEL TODAY: Probably low; this fever has not been seen in recent centuries.

NOTABLE FACT: Sweating sickness was probably what killed Arthur, Prince of Wales, in 1502, freeing up both his wife (Catherine of Aragon) and the path to the throne for his younger brother, Henry VIII.

The first symptom was an ominous feeling of excitement, nervousness, and apprehension.

Other diseases surely came with terror and dread, especially in epidemics when you might hear of deaths across town, then across the street, and then perhaps watch your own family members die. But in the case of the sweating sickness, that nervous feeling was considered a medical symptom. Victims got very little warning, and then the chills began.

The sweat killed quickly. A person might be healthy at lunch, gorging on food and wine, and be dead before dinner. It seemed to punish the gluttonous, mainly striking young and middle-aged men, and more often the upper classes than the lower. Peasants gave it sarcastic names, like the Stop-Gallant.

It seemed to hate the English in particular, not even crossing the border into Wales or Scotland at first. Later, it would visit a few other European countries, but in 1485 this was a disease of England.

It even began with a historic English battle. As the Wars of the Roses were about to end, a nobleman named Thomas, Lord Stanley, apologized to Richard III that his army could not fight in the upcoming battle, since so many were suffering from "the sweat." Then he turned around and offered the same army to Henry Tudor, who won and became King Henry VII.

The army returned to London and was lauded with celebrations by those who were happy to be rid of Richard III. But celebration soon turned to mourning: people began coming down with the sweat. "As it founde them so it toke them, some in sleape some in wake, some in mirthe some in care, some fasting & some ful, some busy and some idle," wrote physician John Caius, who lived through a later outbreak. The sweat struck England five times: in 1485, 1508, 1517, 1528, and 1551.

A FRIGHTFUL EXPERIENCE

Medicine of the 1400s did not know about bacteria or viruses. Doctors treated disease with cures handed down from the ancient physician Galen of Pergamon, or with a guess about how a disease fit in with the theories of the four humors. When the sweating sickness struck, German physician Justus Hecker later wrote, the doctors were completely unprepared. Galen had written nothing about this.

Here is one theory John Caius put together, from the ancient-but-thriving idea of bad air as a cause of disease: The soldiers, even the healthy ones, had unknowingly brought bad air back from the battlefield. When the people of London breathed it in, it overwhelmed their bodies.

The body forces the "evil air" into some part of the body, perhaps the arm or leg, since those are farthest from the vital organs. But if the evil air is plentiful, the infection creeps into the liver, the brain, and the heart. An oppressed heart makes a person want to sleep, and the other impaired body parts dull the senses. The body fights against this "putrefaction venomous" by raising the body's temperature, resulting in the fever, and attempts to sweat out the invading poison.

Most fevers burn for a longer time, writes Caius, like coal or wet wood. But the sweating sickness comes from such a poisonous air that the fever burns up the body extremely fast, never lasting longer than twenty-four hours.

The prevention and cure, he recommended, is to "lyve accordynge to nature" and eat a "pure and cleane diete." Wine is out, peacock meat is in. Salad and fresh fruits may be infected with the evil air, so they should be avoided.

MYSTERY OF THE SWEAT

Whatever struck the English in 1485 seems not to have survived into modern times. After those five outbreaks, it apparently was gone. It may be a virus or bacterium that went extinct, lost forever to history.

But perhaps it survived in a slightly different form. There are diseases we know today with similar symptoms, and it's possible one of these is a relative of the sweating sickness. It's not any of the usual fatal epidemics, like plague or smallpox or typhus, since people of the time would have recognized it as such. The symptoms don't match.

One possibility is relapsing fever, caused by a corkscrew-shaped bacterium that can be spread by ticks or lice. It's called relapsing because the fever lasts a few days, then disappears for about a week. The bacterium then changes its outer coating to disguise itself from the immune system, and can reappear to once again cause sickness.

When relapsing fever is active, symptoms look a lot like the sweat: the patient gets chills and feels agitated and delirious. After this "chill phase," which lasts only about half an hour, comes a "flush phase" with copious sweating. The only problem in matching this up with the English sweat is that relapsing fever often includes a rash or an obvious tick bite. Sweating sickness had neither.

Another theory is hantavirus, which killed twelve people in a 1993 outbreak in the American southwest. The virus was carried by deer mice. Dust from their droppings, if breathed in, caused a disease with sudden, severe shortness of breath. Half of the infected people died.

Hantaviruses occur worldwide, often flying under our radar. Mice can carry them, but so can bats and shrews and voles. A group of Belgian researchers, writing in the journal *Viruses*, argue that hantavirus is a likely cause of sweating sickness, and that rodent droppings can finally explain the centuries-old mystery of why it struck the upper classes harder than the poor.

Everybody had rodents in their houses and farms, but perhaps it was only the rich who tried to keep their houses tidy in spite of the animals. Frequent sweeping could kick up virus-infected dust, making it available for the occupants of the house to breathe in. And that's a situation that no amount of peacock meat can prevent.

CHAPTER 14

THE FIRST INVADERS

INFLUENZA: HISPANIOLA/HAITI
1493

JUST ONE YEAR AFTER CHRISTOPHER COLUMBUS SET FOOT IN NORTH AMERICA, HIS CREW HAD UNLEASHED THE CONTINENT'S FIRST EUROPEAN-DERIVED EPIDEMIC.

DEATH TOLL: Unknown; estimated at 1 million or more

CAUSED BY: Possibly a type of influenza virus

NOTEWORTHY SYMPTOMS: Fever, body aches, runny nose

FATALITY RATE: Unknown, but high

THREAT LEVEL TODAY: Medium. Influenza is a common cause of death among people with weakened immune systems, but epidemics like this one are rare.

NOTABLE FACT: Pigs brought for food may have triggered the epidemic.

B efore Christopher Columbus arrived, millions of Taino people lived on the Caribbean islands, including an island that they called Haiti but which the Spanish named Hispaniola, or at first *La Isla Española*—"the Spanish Island."

Before leaving, Columbus left thirty-eight of his men to build a camp near one of the native villages. He returned the next year with seventeen ships carrying 150 people, and a plan to establish a colony and sail farther to try to find recognizable parts of China. But when he arrived at the previous settlement, it was in ruin: war had broken out between his men and their neighbors, and nobody was left.

Instead, the invaders sailed along the coast and founded a settlement just across from a Taino Indian city on a river. They called it La Isabela, and emptied their ships into it: people, things, and livestock.

Some of that livestock included pigs they had bought on the Canary Islands, a waypoint near Spain. It was December 8. The next day, people began to fall ill. Columbus himself was one of the first. On December 10, he was in bed with a high fever. He didn't write in his diary again until March, suggesting that he wasn't fully recovered until then.

People who had been sent out to explore found they were too sick to continue. Others got sick without leaving the settlement. Soon, according to histories from the time, half of the Spanish were dead as well as countless Taino.

A NEW DISEASE?

Diseases waste little time. When a virus lives amongst people who are used to it, the germ has a tough time: it has to seek out the few susceptible people, dodge their defenses, and make sure its symptoms are mild enough that the victim can walk around and find a new person to gift it to.

Every battle-hardened germ has made compromises as it reaches a semi-truce with the people it lives in and on. Only when a germ makes a sudden leap—for example, as plague did to Europeans—does it have free rein to infect anyone and everyone with as fatal a disease as it likes.

By the time Europeans left for the place they thought was India (which they later called the New World) they were infected by many diseases, and in the centuries to come would share them generously with a population that had none of their defenses. Disease spread early and often beginning in 1492, often catching like fire from one community to another. Some inland cities would have been devastated by European diseases before they ever met a European person.

The Native Americans were probably at a disadvantage due to an accident of genetics. Europeans and Asians have many different HLA proteins, part of the immune system that recognizes invading germs. But the people who then lived all over North and South America were descended from a small group that had arrived over an icy land bridge 15,000 years before. Whatever HLA proteins those people had, those were the ones that the Native Americans of 1492 had in their blood. That explains why they were so hard hit: their bodies didn't recognize they were infected until it was too late.

SWINE FLU?

But the epidemic that hit La Isabela in 1493 killed the Spanish, too. A fatality rate of 50 percent is extreme for almost any disease, so it's likely the people were already weakened from spending a long time at sea and perhaps not having enough food. Their water casks leaked, too.

According to writers of the time, this epidemic also kicked off a massive depopulation of the people who were already living there. Bartolomé de las Casas wrote that "there was so much disease, death, and misery, that innumerable fathers, mothers, and children died . . . Of the multitudes on this island in [1494], by [1506] it was thought there were but one third of all of them left."

After looking over the accounts, medical historian Francisco Guerra believed the epidemic may have been swine flu. The noteworthy symptoms were fever, fatigue, and a high mortality rate; no mention is made of a rash. While smallpox and measles would eventually terrorize the Western Hemisphere, it was not their turn yet.

Instead, it was possibly a form of influenza. Most years, we shrug off "the flu," but the virus mutates unpredictably. Every few years it finds a form that kills people off quicker than usual, and flu pandemics are born. Often they are kicked off from an interspecies shuffling: birds and pigs each have their own form of flu, and new or renewed diseases can be born at this border.

Could this have been what happened in 1493? Swine flu leaping to humans is a rare but possible occurrence. Whatever exactly happened in that epidemic, it would not be the last to result from contact between the "new" and "old" worlds.

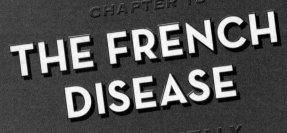

CHAPTER 15

THE FRENCH DISEASE

SYPHILIS: ITALY

1495

HORRIFIC SORES LEADING TO BOUTS OF MADNESS AND EVENTUAL AGONIZING DEATH; IT'S ENOUGH TO MAKE ANYONE STICK TO ABSTINENCE.

DEATH TOLL: Unknown

CAUSED BY: The bacterium *Treponema pallidum*

NOTEWORTHY SYMPTOMS: Gummy tumors that can destroy bone; sores filled with noxious fluid; seizures and dementia; infertility

FATALITY RATE: Unknown

THREAT LEVEL TODAY: Syphilis is less severe today, and can be treated with antibiotics.

NOTABLE FACT: Elaborate wigs may have become popular because syphilis and its treatment, mercury, made so many men go bald.

The Italians called it the French disease; the French called it the Neapolitan disease. In Poland it was the Russian disease. Syphilis was brand new, and nobody wanted to take credit for this affliction, passed from man to woman and back again, that caused horrific sores and eventually sent people to their deaths in bouts of madness.

The French and Italians were, in a sense, both right. The disease first appeared after the French invaded Naples. Both armies were made up of mercenaries recruited from all over the continent, and as the French forces marched toward Naples, they stopped for a month in Rome. At the time, prostitution was one of the amenities that cities offered, and contemporaries said there were more sex workers in Rome than clergy. We can infer how the soldiers spent much of their time.

When they finally left Rome, the forces entered Naples. This was all related to a dispute between the king of Naples, the king of France, and the pope. The details aren't important. The French forces conquered Naples and proceeded to rape and pillage until they were sent home. Shortly afterward, Naples had an outbreak of the mysterious disease. Within a few years, the enemy's disease—whatever name you wanted to use—was widespread. Maybe it came from a Roman brothel, maybe from a victim of war crimes in Naples, or maybe it was carried in from the homeland of one of the mercenaries.

Whatever it was, it was horrible. The German scholar and poet Ulrich von Hutten contracted the disease in the early 1500s, and wrote about dark green boils as big as acorns, filled with a foul stench. The accompanying pain was like being laid on a fire. By the time he wrote the treatise, though, he could report that the disease had changed: not just in his body, because syphilis goes through many stages over the years, but also in the people who were contracting it anew.

The astrologers had predicted that the disease would not endure more than seven years. When its time was up, it persisted, but was milder. The sores were smaller and flatter and there weren't as many of them.

WHAT IS IT AND WHERE DID IT COME FROM?

Hutten described the two theories of his day: The astrologers said the disease came from a blast of evil air that arose from rivers and fields. The physicians, on the other hand, looked for an explanation in their theory of humors. Some imbalance of bodily fluids affected the liver, so that it created bad blood. The blisters were created by blood attempting to leave the body. You knew that the blood was corrupted because when you broke a blister open, the fluid inside was nothing like healthy blood. A doctor and poet named Girolamo Fracastoro coined the name of the disease when he wrote a story in the form of a Greek myth, with the god Apollo cursing a shepherd named Syphilus with sores. The name stuck.

We know today that the disease of syphilis comes from a corkscrew-shaped bacterium called *Treponema pallidum*. If you get syphilis today, the solution is good old penicillin. Still, people don't always seek treatment because it requires admitting what they've been doing: having sex, often with multiple partners.

People figured that out pretty quickly in Hutten's time, too. The disease passed from one person to another, during sexual contact with the open sores. Compatible theories included the idea that people who had the disease were contagious, but also the idea that the disease was a punishment for sinful deeds. Rape would be a sinful deed. Breaking a vow of chastity, if you were a member of the clergy, would be a sinful deed. But for a while, sex within the confines of marriage was not seen as a way to pass on the disease. And so a man who contracted syphilis from a sex worker would not see any problem in having sex with his wife, even if his penis was covered in sores.

LIVING WITH SYPHILIS

The disease was especially hard on women, who often didn't know at first that they had it. The first sign of syphilis in men is often a single sore, called a chancre. In men it may appear on the penis, but in women it's often on the cervix, not visible from outside the body. Today, anyway, it might not hurt and might not itch. It goes away in three to six weeks. The more disastrous symptoms come later.

The secondary stage may involve a fever, and often includes a full body rash. This is when Hutten had his stinking green ulcers. Today, the rash might be small pink or red dots, maybe appearing smeared together, filled with a highly infectious pus.

A woman who contracts the disease may become infertile. If she is pregnant, about half the time she'll miscarry or have a still-born baby. If the baby survives, it has a good chance of being born with syphilis.

The infection lies dormant for years before the third-stage symptoms appear. For an adult, that may mean middle age. At a very young age a child born with syphilis could begin showing signs of the disease, including gummy tumors appropriately called "gumma" that can grow in any tissue, even in bone, even on the face. Medical museums are full of examples of syphilitic skulls, with spongy holes on the forehead where smooth bone should be. If a gumma occurs on the nose, the nose often ends up collapsing.

The disease might fatally infect the aorta, the big artery that comes from the heart to supply the body with blood. It can also infect the brain, leaving the person with seizures or dementia—described at the time as "madness." Syphilis was an undignified way to die.

The disease was so new in 1495 that the doctors were not only baffled by where it came from, but how to treat it. There was no description of anything like it in ancient Greek texts, although some sufferers were probably mistaken for people with other diseases, like leprosy.

One theory at the time was that Columbus had brought it back from the New World. Medical historians still can't decide if that theory is true. Syphilis's first rampages in Europe were so soon after the voyage that the timeline seems unlikely. And no disease quite like syphilis existed in the New World either.

We know, though, that there are other diseases in the world that are *like* syphilis. Yaws is one; it produces similar symptoms but is not sexually transmitted. Perhaps it was yaws that sailed back on Columbus's ship, and the little corkscrew took advantage of its new environment and fresh population to evolve into something nobody had ever seen before.

Whatever its route, syphilis was a game-changer. Nations and churches dragged sexuality into their wars and arguments, since allegedly celibate priests were often marked for life. And eventually the disease was so widespread that there was no point in blaming it on another country. England demoted the long-standing "pox" to "small pox" and called the once-new disease "great pox." Elsewhere, people just called it syphilis.

CHAPTER 16

THE DANCING PLAGUE

MASS PSYCHOGENIC ILLNESS: STRASBOURG

1518

THIS IS JUST WHAT IT SOUNDS LIKE: PEOPLE DANCED UNTIL THEY DIED OF EXHAUSTION. INSTEAD OF A VIRUS OR PARASITE, THE CAUSE OF THIS ONE WAS ALL IN THEIR HEADS.

DEATH TOLL: Unknown; at least dozens

CAUSED BY: Mass psychogenic illness involving a trance-like state

NOTEWORTHY SYMPTOMS: Dancing, exhaustion

FATALITY RATE: Unknown

THREAT LEVEL TODAY: Low

NOTABLE FACT: There have been many dancing plagues throughout history, recorded as early as the seventh century and as late as 1863. Most occurred in an area surrounding the Rhine River between modern-day France and Germany.

Frau Troffea was the first. She began dancing, one story goes, to make a fool of her husband, and encouraged other women to do the same. But when they began to dance, they found that they could not stop. This was the beginning of a deadly epidemic of dancing that struck Strasbourg, in what is now France, in 1518.

The dancing plague's origin story sounds far-fetched, but the plague itself was real. The dancing was contagious: it began with one person and spread to her neighbors, and by the end of the summer hundreds of people were afflicted. The city's council consulted doctors to figure out how to stop the dance from spreading.

Our best understanding, looking back through the years, is that the dancing plague was a mass psychogenic illness, and that the dancers were in a trance state, oblivious to the outside world and perhaps unable to feel pain. Trances like this are real, and so is the idea that an imaginary disease can spread like a real one, with its victims believing fully that they are sick or supernaturally possessed.

Many cultures have rituals involving trances. Before entering the trance state, people know what to expect: how long a trance should last, and what people do while in a trance. The San people of southern Africa dance with rhythmic steps when participating in healing trance ceremonies. Protestants in the American South would scream and faint during prayer meetings. And the people of Strasbourg, knowing their region had a history of dancing plagues stretching back hundreds of years, picked up their feet and danced.

SETTING THE STAGE

The decades leading up to the epidemic were fraught with terror and strife. John Waller, in *The Dancing Plague: The Strange, True Story of an Extraordinary Illness*, lists a series of events that left residents of the region fearing for their souls. In 1492, a meteor struck near Strasbourg. In 1495, conjoined twins were born, baby boys joined at the forehead. In the following years, plague and famine struck repeatedly. Syphilis appeared, and seemed to be God's punishment for adultery and fornication.

Over and over harvests failed, vegetables froze in the ground, families were forced to slaughter animals they couldn't feed. Looking for scapegoats, they attacked Jews and Gypsies. Three times Bundschuh was attempted, a bloody peasants' revolt that some saw as expressing a divine right to resist oppression. Just before the dancing plague began, in 1517, crops froze in the fields and hailstorms finished off what was left. Loans from previous years came due. This was the year that, amid many bad years, one chronicler called "the bad year." People appealed to the clergy to ask for God's mercy but masses, prayers, and processions did nothing to relieve their suffering.

The people of Strasbourg surely knew of the many dancing plagues that had come before. In 1347, a series of them had spread along the rivers that wander between modern-day Netherlands, Germany, France, Belgium, Luxembourg, and Switzerland. In town after town, people took up the dance, leaping and running while screaming in pain. They called on God and saints to help them, and bystanders wrote that the people were possessed by demons. A century earlier, in the town of Erfurt, a story tells of a hundred children that danced out of town on the feast day of St. Vitus.

Today, "St. Vitus's dance" is the nickname of a seizure-like disorder called Sydenham's chorea. But at the time, St. Vitus was known for both curing and causing uncontrollable dancing, as well as seizures (and, because a saint might as well diversify, infertility in women). The dancers of 1518, it is clear from eyewitness accounts, were not falling down and suffering from seizures. They were on their feet, dancing with painful abandon.

CURING THE PLAGUE

Six days after Frau Troffea began her dance, the local lord ordered that she be taken thirty miles away to Saverne, where a shrine to St. Vitus stood at the top of a small mountain. We have no record of whether she made it there, or whether she was cured. The contagion spread in her absence: thirty-four dancers after the first week, fifty after just eleven days. Eventually they numbered in the hundreds, dancing day and night in sweat-soaked clothes and bloody shoes.

Strasbourg's city council discussed the need to end this epidemic before it got any worse. Determined to take a scientific approach, they consulted the physicians' guild rather than turning to the clergy. The physicians' state-of-the-art medical knowledge allowed them to decree that the dancing was a disease caused by overheated blood.

The cure, they said, was to encourage the dancing. So the council ordered the carpenters' and tanners' guilds to convert their buildings to dancehalls. They ordered that a grain market be likewise cleared out, and led dancers into this area too. Finally, they hired builders to construct a stage in a field normally used as a horse-trading market, and hired musicians to play for the dancers, mainly on flutes and drums.

The afflicted were not alone. The guild members and dancers' families were told to join in, to keep the dancers from hurting themselves and to encourage them to keep dancing. Anyone who fell down was goaded to get back up. Occasionally a dancer would recover from the trance, only to immediately relapse. Since we know that mass psychogenic illness is shaped by suggestion, putting the dancers on a public stage and encouraging others to join in was probably not helping to end the epidemic. But this approach continued until people started dying.

The council then changed tactics. The stage was torn down, the crowds dispersed. Musicians were sent home. Families were told to keep dancers in their homes, away from public view. The city temporarily banished "loose persons," including sex workers and gamblers. Any sort of dancing was banned for the next two months, unless it was done by "honorable persons" in their homes, and then only if the music was provided by stringed instruments, never by drums.

What finally ended the outbreak was a journey to the faraway shrine of St. Vitus. The afflicted were herded onto wagons and taken to the chapel for a special mass. The sufferers were walked around the altar, and required to donate a penny to the church. They were also given a precious gift: red shoes that were blessed with holy water and oil. Shoes were valuable; red dyes were some of the most expensive on the market. The color may have represented blood, or the flames under the martyred St. Vitus.

The sufferers went home, and the plague died down. The next three years brought good harvests, and Martin Luther's Protestantism gave people an outlet for their distrust of the Catholic Church. Supernatural afflictions fell out of favor as science became more fashionable, and Europe never saw another dancing plague.

CHAPTER 17

THE FALL OF MOCTEZUMA

SMALLPOX: TENOCHTITLÁN
1520

THE SPANISH CONQUISTADORS HAD MANY WEAPONS ON THEIR SIDE WHEN THEY INVADED TENOCHTITLÁN: HORSES, GUNS, AND SWORDS WERE THE OBVIOUS ONES. BUT ONE OF THE MOST INSTRUMENTAL WEAPONS WAS AN INVISIBLE ONE, BROUGHT BY ACCIDENT: SMALLPOX.

DEATH TOLL: Estimated at 240,000

CAUSED BY: The smallpox virus *Variola major*

NOTEWORTHY SYMPTOMS: Fever and a rash of pustules

FATALITY RATE: Estimated at 40 percent

THREAT LEVEL TODAY: Gone. Smallpox has been eradicated.

NOTABLE FACT: Before the Spanish arrived, Tenochtitlán was bigger than most cities in Europe.

A frenzy of sailing followed Columbus's voyages. Ships criss-crossed the Atlantic bringing gold and goods, plants and food, slaves and adventure-seekers, often terror and bloodshed. Disease, of course, was not left behind.

Syphilis was probably the only disease to travel from west to east, but plenty went the other way. Influenza, malaria, yellow fever, and measles all showed up early in the game. There was an epidemic among the Guanche people that the Spanish named "Guanche drowsiness." The people were soon enslaved, and by 1600 they were gone. Meanwhile plague sputtered through Europe, typhus broke out here and there, and a few outbreaks of what may have been smallpox occurred on Caribbean islands.

The Europeans watched and wrote as diseases wiped out whole Native American villages, or left them too weak to resist takeovers. They scrapped plans to turn the natives into slaves, and instead began importing captive Africans. The new slaves' diseases entered the mix.

Somewhere, someone brought smallpox. The terrifying virus probably sparked a few small epidemics before catching like fire on Hispaniola (now Haiti and Dominican Republic). From there it hopped to Cuba and Costa Rica. For some reason it didn't catch on in North America until later. But in 1519 the virus disembarked on the shores of what is now Mexico. There, it assisted in one of the Spanish conquistadors' bloodiest battles.

A PLAN

Hernán Cortés began collecting men and outfitting ships under a short-lived order from the governor of Cuba to look for gold and other riches and report back. The governor must have gotten wind of Cortés's actual plans, because he sent a messenger to cancel the trip. According to legend, the messenger got to the port just in time to see Cortés's ships pulling away. Their cargo: 550 soldiers, sixteen horses, and a few guns.

On the mainland in what is today Mexico, Cortés established a town, stepped down from his post as captain, and had the men elect him as governor. Then he burned their ships to remove the possibility of retreat. Their goal: the city of Tenochtitlán in the Mexica empire, reputed to be huge and gleaming with treasure.

At first, the men fought against the people of Tlaxcala. Cortés's force won every battle, probably thanks to horses and weaponry, but lost men every time. Soon he realized that the four kingdoms of Tlaxcala were enemies of the Mexica, and that the Mexica had plenty of other enemies. The kings of Tlaxcala agreed to attack the city with Cortés, probably figuring they could beat the Spanish in an all-out battle if it came to that.

Cortés was leading an army of 20,000 when he reached Tenochtitlán. It was a city bigger than Paris, built on artificial islands in the middle of a mountain lake. It had aqueducts, clean streets laid out in a grid pattern, markets, palaces, floating gardens. There was nothing like it in Spain.

The emperor, Moctezuma, was afraid something like this might happen—but he was expecting some sort of attack from the gods, foretold by omens years earlier. So he welcomed the invaders, who entered his palace and took him captive. Months passed.

A DECISIVE VICTORY

Meanwhile, the deciding factor was ready to make its entrance. A ship sent by the Cuban governor had landed with orders to arrest Cortés. The conquistador, warned by allies near the coast, took some of his men to meet them. He captured the ship's leader and added the rest of the men to his own small army. But on that ship was a slave named Francisco Baguía, who had smallpox. The virus returned to Tenochtitlán with Cortés's crew.

In his absence, the Mexica had arrested the Spaniards who had stayed behind. Moctezuma now begged his people to spare the Spanish. Then Moctezuma was killed. The Spanish said the Mexica killed him, and the Mexica said the opposite. Moctezuma's son Cuitláhuac became the new emperor and drove the Spanish out of the city in a hail of arrows, leaving 600 bodies behind—at least one of them infected with smallpox. The Mexica even destroyed the bridge to the mainland to trap the conquistadors, who managed to escape by walking on piles of their dead compatriots.

Smallpox had entered the palace, and was now ready to do the real conquering. Cuitláhuac only ruled for four months before he died of the disease. Cortés intended to make friends with more of the Mexica's enemies, but found this almost too easy: several local kingdoms had lost leaders to smallpox, and Cortés found ways to step in. He attacked Tenochtitlán for the last time in 1521, when the city had lost at least a third of its population. Another 100,000 people died in the battle, still considered one of the bloodiest in history.

Smallpox was not done; it spread through the rest of Mexica territory, and onward. It created a sequel to this story 3,000 miles south, when the epidemic killed the Inca king and his heir, weakening the kingdom so that Francisco Pizarro could take over. Within a hundred years, it reached Massachusetts. Smallpox would continue terrorizing the people of the Americas for many years to come, natives and newcomers alike.

CHAPTER 18

THE LOST CURE FOR SCURVY

SCURVY: STADACONA (MODERN-DAY QUEBEC)
— 1536 —

IT WOULD BE HUNDREDS OF YEARS BEFORE PEOPLE WOULD REALLY UNDERSTAND WHAT CAUSED SCURVY. BUT IN THE FROZEN CANADIAN WINTER, ONE SHIP CAPTAIN LEARNED OF A SURE-FIRE CURE—PINE NEEDLES.

DEATH TOLL: 25 out of a crew of 110

CAUSED BY: Deficiency of vitamin C

NOTEWORTHY SYMPTOMS: Swollen and gangrenous flesh, including the gums

FATALITY RATE: 100 percent if untreated

THREAT LEVEL TODAY: Low

NOTABLE FACT: Citrus fruit isn't your only option to fight scurvy! Apple cider and a plant called "scurvy grass" have enough vitamin C to stave off the dreaded disease.

L ost teeth were the least of their worries.

The sailors on Jacques Cartier's second expedition, the one that got as far into Canada as modern-day Quebec City, were dying in their ship. They had set sail from Saint-Malo in France, and calculated that the winter in their destination would be warm and mild. So they were utterly unprepared when it turned out to be frigid, and the ice froze around their boat.

The men suffered that winter from scurvy, probably in addition to other diseases and deficiencies. Their captain wrote that the men lost all their strength. Their legs swelled; tendons contracted and turned black as coal. The flesh of their gums swelled and rotted, and yes, their teeth sometimes fell out. Cartier ordered that one of the corpses be cut open, revealing rotten organs and pools of dark blood.

The explorer and his men had no way of knowing that the disease came from a lack of vitamin C in their diet. Instead, they guessed they had somehow caught it from the Native Americans in the nearby Iroquois town of Stadacona, some of whom had fallen ill around the same time.

One day Cartier recognized an Iroquois man who had been sick just a few weeks before, and casually asked if there was a treatment for the disease, since he had a servant on the ship who was sick. (In reality, he had recorded that "of the 110 men forming our company, there were not ten in good health . . .") The Native Americans taught him how to gather and boil the branches of a tree whose name Cartier recorded as *annedda*.

At first, the French sailors were suspicious of the brew. When they tried it, and found that it cured their scurvy, they went and cut down an entire tree. The ship's chronicler wrote that "all the drugs of Alexandria . . . could not have done so much in a year as did this tree in eight days." According to that record, it cured every disease the sailors had, including syphilis. (More likely, the sailors found having syphilis alone a relief after living with syphilis plus scurvy.)

We don't know for sure what the annedda tree was. It may have been the eastern white pine, the balsam fir, the arborvitae, the

black spruce, or the white hemlock, to name a few modern bota-
nists' guesses. From the Europeans' perspective, a scurvy cure was
found and lost—and not for the last time.

SCIENCE TO THE RESCUE (SORT OF)

Over the years, many scurvy cures were proposed. Some were
effective, some not, and it was hard to tell the difference between
them. For example, several experts said that fresh fruits and vegetables were necessary to prevent scurvy; however, some vegetables
contain lots of vitamin C while others contain little. Broccoli has
plenty, for example, but dried peas (more common on ships' voyages) have next to none.

What's worse, attempts to keep the cures fresh on a ship's voyage backfired. An herb called "scurvy grass" has as much vitamin C
as orange juice when it's fresh. So crews dried the herb to make tea
from it while at sea, but drying and storing it destroyed the vitamin
C content.

Dozens of scurvy cures each had their own champions when
James Lind, surgeon on the HMS *Salisbury* in 1747, decided to
answer the question once and for all. He waited until the men
began developing scurvy, and then conducted an experiment
on twelve of them. Two sick sailors were given citrus fruit daily
with their rations. Another pair tried each of the other proposed
cures: cider, vinegar, elixir of vitriol (basically, a weak solution of
acid), a medicinal paste made of spices, and a regimen of saltwater
laxatives.

The experiment was short-lived, because Lind ran out of oranges
and lemons after just six days. But the men who had eaten the fruit
were then well enough to work again and take care of the others.
The men who drank the cider had improved slightly, and nobody
else had fared as well. Lind wrote up his results in 1753, after years
of further research, but because so little was known about vitamin
deficiencies and because Lind himself misunderstood his results,
scurvy remained a mystery.

UNDERSTANDING SCURVY

People had been suffering from vitamin deficiencies since time immemorial. In years of famine, in sieges on cities, in harsh winters, scurvy and other diseases would plague communities. But vitamin deficiencies were no better understood than other diseases. In fact, they looked similar, striking people who lived together, ate the same food, breathed the same air, and rubbed dirty shoulders with each other.

James Lind concluded that sailors' body fluids, or humors, rotted in their bodies, and that acid could stop this rotting. Citrus fruit worked because it was acidic. He couldn't explain why the other acidic cures didn't. For some reason, the idea of an essential nutrient sounded less believable than the idea that fluids could rot inside your body and would poison you if you didn't sweat them out.

Lind's other ideas were right. He said that it was bad for sailors' health to live crowded together, to eat moldy biscuits and rotten meat (the staples of the diet on a long voyage), and that infectious diseases could run rampant in a weakened population. He didn't catch that the sailors were usually vitamin deficient even at the start of a voyage and that their bodies' frequent dealings with infection and injury meant that they needed vitamin C even more than the average peasant or farmer.

The idea was so hard to suss out that vitamin C was not discovered until the 1930s. Vitamins A and B had recently been discovered, so the idea was on scientists' minds when guinea pigs in their lab showed signs of scurvy when placed on a minimal diet. Scurvy was once thought to be purely a human disease, but we share a quirk with guinea pigs, fruit bats, and some primates: while most other mammals make their own vitamin C, we need to get it in our diet.

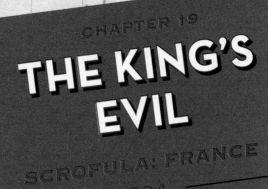

CHAPTER 19

THE KING'S EVIL

SCROFULA: FRANCE
1594

SUFFERING FROM A LUMPY, SWOLLEN, PAINFUL NECK? DON'T WORRY, YOUR LOCAL KING CAN CURE YOU.

DEATH TOLL: Unknown

CAUSED BY: The bacterium *Mycobacterium tuberculosis*

NOTEWORTHY SYMPTOMS: Swollen lymph nodes in the neck, sometimes developing ulcers

FATALITY RATE: Swollen lymph nodes by themselves are not fatal, but can progress into a more dangerous version of tuberculosis

THREAT LEVEL TODAY: Low. Scrofula can be treated with antibiotics.

NOTABLE FACT: Samuel Johnson, the famous dictionary writer, had scrofula as a child and was taken to England to be touched by Queen Anne. The belief at the time was that the touch of a ruler would cure the disease (it did not).

If you were crowned king of France, what would be the first thing on your to-do list? For Henry IV, who took the throne in 1594, curing scrofula was item number one.

The king's physician recorded that Henry IV healed 1,500 people after his coronation. He knelt at the hospital of St. Marcoul in Corbeny and made the sign of the cross over each person's head, saying (in French), "The king touches thee, may God heal thee."

Scrofula was a form of tuberculosis, better known as a lung disease—but tuberculosis is no one-trick pony. In medieval Europe, one of its better-known forms was an infection of the lymph nodes in the neck, then called scrofula—or the King's Evil. That doesn't mean, of course, that the king did something evil to afflict you with it. The term was used more broadly for dreaded diseases. Epilepsy was known for a time as the "falling evil," evoking the oh-crap moment of being overtaken by a seizure while you're out for a walk.

The king earned his association with scrofula by his role in *curing* the disease. If you had a lumpy, swollen neck, you took yourself—or your parents would take you—to the monarch of France or England. This person had the power to cure you.

The healing powers were said to trace back to the first French king, Clovis I, who united the Frankish tribes in a series of conquests. In the midst of this war, he converted to Catholicism. The priest charged with bringing the sacred oil for his baptism was running late, so a dove flew down from heaven with a special batch. This "holy phial" was then used to anoint each king after Clovis as well, and represented a special divine blessing.

At least that was the explanation given centuries later to explain why royalty should have the power to cure disease. People had been flocking to the king to cure their various illnesses, and somewhere along the line scrofula became known as a royal specialty.

THE ROYAL TOUCH

Scrofula represents an ongoing battle between *Mycobacterium tuberculosis* and a person's immune system. Some days the germ wins, some days it loses. Eventually, the immune system may get the infection under control. Because of this back and forth, people who are touched by the king may find that their scrofula goes away. This coincidence could be credited to the king's divine powers. (People who asked the king to cure, for example, leprosy would not be so lucky.) This is probably how the king's touch got its reputation. (If the king's touch didn't work, you could try surgery, which is what Samuel Johnson ended up needing.)

Lymph nodes are part of a system that collects immune system cells from throughout the body, plus sometimes bits of the invaders they're fighting. We have about 450 lymph nodes scattered around our body: some in the groin, some in the armpits, and some deep inside our chest, to name a few. The lymph nodes under your jawline swell when you get a cold. The buboes of bubonic plague are another type of swollen lymph nodes. And the lymph nodes running along both sides of the neck are a popular destination for tuberculosis bacteria.

These lymph nodes swell, painlessly at first, but on the inside they can become full of pus and dead tissue. The immune system tries to wall off the infection with scar tissue, but sometimes it bursts. The result can be purplish stains on the skin, or open sores. When tuberculosis bacteria were roaming through medieval populations, scrofula was a sadly common sight, especially in children.

The roots of the touching ritual were buried in legend, but they evolved from an occasional thing to a formal event. According to legend, the healing power given to Philip I of France disappeared due to his sinful conduct. He made a pilgrimage to Corbeny where relics of St. Marcoul helped him regain the healing touch, and afterward reportedly cured sufferers by the hundreds at that same church.

Rulers of the time were expected to show their love for the people by helping the poor, and in time the ritual came to include a gift of money. After delivering his healing touch, the king would direct an assistant to give the scrofulous person a coin, often punched in the middle so it could be worn on a ribbon.

Historians have suggested that the king's touch was the most popular during times when royalty felt threatened (by the church or by political enemies) and wanted to show that they were very special people, endorsed by God. Later, English people started asking their king to touch for scrofula too.

The gold coins probably didn't hurt the ritual's popularity, either. Eventually sufferers would need a royal certificate to receive their blessing and gold coin; to get the certificate they had to be examined to make sure they actually had scrofula.

The tradition began to die out in the 1700s. Scrofula itself was becoming less common (it would ebb and flow over the centuries), but people were also beginning to be more interested in scientific rather than supernatural explanations of things like disease. The days of counting on a miracle were over.

CHAPTER 20

SQUANTO'S BACKSTORY

UNKNOWN DISEASE: MASSACHUSETTS

1616

THE NATIVE AMERICANS AT THE FIRST THANKSGIVING WEREN'T DISINTERESTED BYSTANDERS; THEY WERE STRATEGIZING TO SURVIVE IN A WORLD TURNED UPSIDE DOWN BY DISEASE.

DEATH TOLL: Estimated at 20,000

CAUSED BY: Unknown

NOTEWORTHY SYMPTOMS: Headache, fever, and yellowed skin

FATALITY RATE: Estimated at 90 percent

THREAT LEVEL TODAY: Unknown

NOTABLE FACT: Tisquantum—who you probably know as Squanto—only escaped the epidemic because he was taken to Europe as a captive.

S top me if you've heard this one: A group of English families makes a deadly voyage, losing half their members to famine and disease once they drop anchor in what is now Massachusetts. They are saved, though, by a friendly Native American named Squanto, beginning a friendly relationship between the Pilgrims and the locals. Both factions live peacefully side by side, even sharing a harvest celebration at the end of that first year. In other words, it's the story of the first Thanksgiving.

Colonists and Native Americans keeping peace for years is indeed an accomplishment. But this heartwarming tale has a little more to it. How did the Pilgrims survive that first winter without Squanto? Why was Squanto so eager to help them, anyway? The answer lies in an epidemic.

Let's rewind to 1614, six years before the Pilgrims' arrival. There was not yet a town called Plymouth, but in its spot on the map was a Native American village called Patuxet. John Smith (of Pocahontas fame) came there with two ships intending to hunt whales. When that was unsuccessful, he switched his crews to fishing and fur trading. When he came to Patuxet territory, the locals gave him a tour of their gardens and orchards. Soon afterward, Smith left for England, and his second-in-command invited the Patuxet to visit the remaining ship. The sailors shoved the Native Americans into the hold, slaughtering any that resisted. Twenty survivors were taken to Spain to be sold as slaves. One of them was a warrior-bodyguard known as Tisquantum—later nicknamed Squanto.

Spanish clergy stopped the sale and freed the slaves. Tisquantum traveled to London, where he stayed with a shipbuilder who had investments in North America. Tisquantum learned to speak English during his stay, and eventually talked his host into getting him on a ship to Newfoundland—still over a thousand miles from home, but at least on the right continent.

In the meantime, the Patuxet and neighboring communities swore off any more friendly contact with intruders. When a French ship wrecked at Cape Cod, they killed most of the crew and took five survivors captive. It seemed that Europeans, even harmless-looking ones, would never be welcomed.

SQUANTO RETURNS

From the Newfoundland fishing village where he was working, Tisquantum talked an explorer into setting out for Patuxet, with himself as interpreter and guide. In 1619, Tisquantum finally returned home. But his home was gone.

Two hundred miles of coastline, formerly full of busy villages, were now completely deserted. Fields were overgrown, houses were falling down, and skeletons were scattered among them. Tisquantum's village was part of the devastation. When they finally found a few surviving families, the survivors sent for Massasoit, leader of the Wampanoag. He arrived with one of the shipwrecked French sailors, who explained the situation. Here's how merchant Thomas Morton later described it:

> "[The sailor] had learned so much of [his Nauset captors'] language as to rebuke them for their bloudy deede, saying that God would be angry with them for it, and that hee would in his displeasure destroy them; but the Salvages (it seemes boasting of their strength) replyd and sayd, that they were so many that God could not kill them."

Many of the Nauset were killed anyway, in the epidemic that followed. The English were happy to credit the slaughter to God, as a sign that the Pilgrims were meant to take the land. Estimates put the dead at about 90 percent of the area's native population. Several groups went extinct.

Tisquantum ended up as Massasoit's captive. He talked up the advantages of siding with the English, essentially using the Pilgrims as a pawn in a complex political situation that pitted Massasoit's Wampanoag nation, weakened with the loss of so many people to disease, against stronger enemies surrounding them. The alliance could help the Wampanoag, Tisquantum argued, while in the process elevating Tisquantum from prisoner to valuable translator.

When the Pilgrims arrived, they built their new settlement on the site of Tisquantum's former home. The Wampanoag watched and waited. Eventually Massasoit gave his blessing for Tisquantum to speak to the English. They helped the Pilgrims to get their farming endeavors off the ground (although the Pilgrims had been raiding abandoned villages for food and goods), and had them sign a treaty stating that the Pilgrims and Wampanoag would each defend the other if needed. An uneasy peace followed for an amazing fifty years. Tisquantum didn't live to see it, though. He died after two years, shortly after Massasoit threatened to execute him as a traitor (long story). But Tisquantum was not killed in battle or executed. He died of disease, one that seemed familiar to the English who wrote that he suffered from the "Indian fever." It was probably the same disease that had wiped out his village.

INDIAN FEVER

It's not clear what the disease was that killed so many people. One clue is its Native American name, which refers to the color yellow. Witnesses described the disease as giving people's skin a yellow hue. One interpretation is that this is the yellowish pus color of smallpox pustules, which can run together into giant masses of pus covering patches of skin.

But a number of diseases can give the skin a true yellow tinge—this symptom is known as jaundice, and it can happen when a disease affects the liver. Yellow fever is one; malaria can do the same. Hepatitis, which can be carried by several viruses, is also a possibility.

Another convincing hypothesis is leptospirosis, caused by a corkscrew-shaped bacterium that is a distant relative of Lyme disease and syphilis. This bacterium is carried by rodents, and often transmitted when people step into contaminated water. The English remarked on the Native Americans' odd habit of bathing—at the time, many Europeans didn't. Wading barefoot in water could have passed the disease around, if it really was leptospirosis. The theory is especially attractive because sometimes leptospirosis infections can cause a condition called Weil's disease. The two most notable symptoms are jaundice (yellow skin) and a tendency toward nosebleeds. "Indian fever" was known to include both. Whatever the cause, New England would never be the same again.

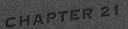

CHAPTER 21

THE FIRST MIRACLE CURE

MALARIA: PERU

1630

MALARIA QUICKLY FOUND A HOME IN SOUTH AMERICA. BUT ITS REIGN OF TERROR WOULD NOT LAST LONG—SOON THE WORLD HAD A MIRACULOUS MALARIA CURE.

DEATH TOLL: Unknown; millions

CAUSED BY: Mosquito-borne *Plasmodium* parasites

NOTEWORTHY SYMPTOMS: Chills and a fever that recurs every few days

FATALITY RATE: Unknown; today the fatality rate is less than 1 percent

THREAT LEVEL TODAY: High in many parts of the world

NOTABLE FACT: Quinine is thought to be the first-ever pharmaceutical treatment, because it kills a specific pathogen, rather than just helping symptoms.

Malaria racked the New World just as it had the old. It stowed away in the blood of newcomers, both the Europeans who invaded and then settled, and the Africans they enslaved.

In those days, malaria was not a tropical disease. Its origins may have been in Africa, but the microscopic parasite had long before blanketed Europe's and Asia's swampy areas. When ships set off from Europe full of entrepreneurs and pilgrims and adventurers and settlers, they were leaving from some of the most malaria-ridden places on the continent. Among the Jamestown settlers whose birthplaces are known, more than half came from the marshy areas whose populations had high rates of something they called "ague."

There was no specific word for the parasite or for the disease it caused. The medical language of the time had words for bad air arising from swamps, like "miasma" and, yes, "malaria," and there were words for fever and chills. Many illnesses cause fevers, so at first it would seem impossible to tell when anybody was talking about malaria versus any of hundreds of other diseases.

Except that malaria's fever runs an unusual course. It's triggered when the parasites emerge from red blood cells, and subsides when they hide again. The ancient Greeks wrote about a cycle in which a person would have a sudden attack of chills, followed by fever, on the first day. The second day brought relief. The third day would start another attack. This was known as a "tertian," or third-day fever, and the attacks could continue every other day for weeks at a time.

This is the ague, meaning "acute": a strong, sudden attack of chills. (Sometimes ague referred to the chills; sometimes to the cyclical ailment as a whole.) Besides the tertian fever or ague, there was also a quartan version, repeating on the fourth instead of third day.

One of Columbus's men came down with something like ague, but that could have been a fever due to swine flu or anything else. But before long, people all over the Western Hemisphere were writing back home about their tertian and quartan fevers. Malaria was surely one of the diseases that sickened Native Americans, and it wasn't kind to Europeans either. People who stepped off a boat had a one-in-three chance of dying their first year; those who got the ague and survived were considered to be "seasoned." Africans were often immune.

Recurring fevers were a problem throughout the Americas, although Europeans back home were also plagued with them. What people needed most was something they did not realize even existed: a cure for this disease. They had "cures," of course, or treatments. Most were not effective. Bloodletting, for example, was a standard treatment, to help the patient's body get rid of the poison that was supposedly building up in the blood to cause the fever.

Other treatments tended toward the spiritual. One sixteenth-century remedy involved writing the the made-up mystical word "Abracolam" over and over with letters missing, until finally you just wrote the letter "A." This scrap of paper would then be tied to your neck by a virgin while she recited three Our Father prayers and three Hail Mary prayers. But even as people ventured farther from malaria's original birthplace in Africa, they found themselves closer to an amazing thing: a specific, pharmaceutical cure.

THE PHARMACY

Native Americans and Europeans each had their own herbal remedies—some helpful for specific symptoms, many not. Nobody yet had a plant that would cure a specific disease, killing the organism that caused it. That makes sense, since it would be hundreds of years before the idea of germs would take hold: a fever was just a thing the body did when its humors were upset by the stench of swampy air.

Among the many ships that set sail for the Americas were some that were full of Jesuits, an order of Catholic priests and brothers. The Jesuits' plan in South America was to have their priests live among the native people, learn their language, and attempt to win them over to Christianity. In the meantime, one of the priests made it his mission to establish a pharmacy—not just for the local community, but one that could supply the other Jesuit missions in the area. These two plans clicked together when, one day, a Jesuit apothecary gave a fever sufferer a warm cup of bark tea.

There was a very specific tree that this bark came from, one with green leaves that would turn red on the underside, and that produced tufts of pink trumpet-shaped flowers in summer. Some of the bark of this tree, dried into powder, was a favorite of the locals for anyone shivering from cold. If you had been swimming in a cold river, or came home near-freezing and covered in snow, a cup of tea made from this bark would ease your shivers. That's because the bark's active ingredient, quinine, is a muscle relaxant.

Agustino Salumbrino, the priest who ran the pharmacy in Lima, gave a cup of this tea to a Jesuit brother suffering from the chills of ague. To his surprise it not only quieted the chills, but also stopped the fevers from recurring. The priests asked the locals for more information about this plant. The Peruvians taught the Jesuits how to take the bark from the tree in vertical strips, to avoid killing it, and told them that for every tree they cut down, they should plant five more. Not surprisingly, the priests made their plantings in the shape of a cross.

They didn't know why it worked, just that it did. Even today we aren't totally sure why. It seems to stop the malaria parasite, which lives inside red blood cells, from being able to fully digest the hemoglobin it eats. The parasite is poisoned from within.

A mythology sprung up around the mysterious bark. An Italian doctor made up a story about a Spanish countess who was cured by it in Lima. The Countess of Chinchón was a real person, though, and the tree became known as *cinchona*. The Peruvian Indians' word for the tree, *quinquina*, eventually lent its name to the active ingredient, quinine.

But even from this early beginning, there were problems. *Quinquina* referred to more than one type of tree, and not all of them had quinine in the bark. If a collector got the wrong kind, or harvested it at the wrong time of year, or if somewhere along the line it was mixed with other ingredients, the finished medicine that went into an ague sufferer's mouth could be anything from a strong to a completely useless drug. Some people swore by the powder, and some scoffed at it.

The miracle cure didn't save many lives, at least at first. It was expensive and the association with Jesuits was unfashionable in many corners: Jesuits were Catholic, and Protestantism was the hot new thing. Archduke Leopold of Austria, governor of the Low Countries, came down with a quartan fever and grudgingly took cinchona. When his fever came back a month later, he ordered his physician to write a treatise, "Exposé of the Febrifuge Powder from the American World," declaring its uselessness.

Meanwhile in England, those who didn't want cinchona could buy another supposed miracle cure, called "Talbor's Wonderful Secret." Its creator warned people away from Jesuits' powder, saying that it was dangerous and that only his secret cure was safe and effective. Robert Talbor used his elixir to cure King Charles II of England, who later sent Talbor to his friend Louis XIV of France when that king's last surviving son became ill. Delighted, the French king paid Talbor for the recipe, agreeing not to reveal it until Talbor's death. It turned out to be opium, wine, and cinchona.

Talbor had, in fact, been buying up all the best-quality bark so that his competitors couldn't get it. It really was a miracle cure if you could get a strong enough dose, and in time people realized that—especially the countries invested in imperialism. For them, giving quinine to an officer or worker in America or Africa was essentially giving that person the power to defy death.

Countries feuded over who could have the best quinine, and who could have it at all. Bolivia began to limit the number of people who were allowed to collect and sell it; enterprising traders smuggled the seeds out of the country. For years, the drug was too expensive to give in large quantities to everybody who needed it. Eventually, synthetic versions of quinine and of the Chinese herb artimesia (rediscovered from ancient medical texts) hit the market. Today, malaria is still hard to control, but now at least we have a few drugs to work with.

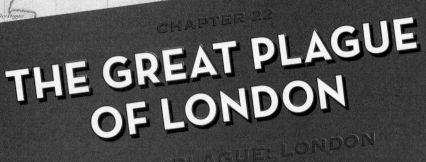

CHAPTER 22

THE GREAT PLAGUE OF LONDON

BUBONIC PLAGUE: LONDON

1665

PLAGUE WASN'T FINISHED AFTER THE BLACK DEATH; IT MADE COMEBACKS FOR CENTURIES, INCLUDING THIS MASSIVE OUTBREAK IN LONDON.

DEATH TOLL: Estimated at 100,000

CAUSED BY: The bacterium *Yersinia pestis*

NOTEWORTHY SYMPTOMS: Swollen lymph nodes ("buboes") in groin, armpits, or neck

FATALITY RATE: Unknown, but 60 percent is typical for bubonic plague

THREAT LEVEL TODAY: Low. Plague is rare, and can be treated with antibiotics if caught in time.

NOTABLE FACT: Isaac Newton was among the people who left town during the plague. He invented calculus over the following years while staying in the countryside.

The first death was unremarkable. A woman in one of London's outlying parishes, St. Giles-in-the-Fields, died of plague on Christmas Eve in 1664.

Ever since the Black Death had swept the continent centuries before, plague had never really disappeared. The disease would visit in small epidemics every few years, often seeming to target children who hadn't been around to develop an immunity to it the previous time. Most years had at least a few plague deaths, maybe a poor family or two and the people who inherited their unwashed clothes and mattresses.

The next plague death wasn't until February 1665; after that, not until April. But eventually, London city officials began to wonder if the records were correct. The city published "Bills of Mortality" that included causes of death, and in 1665 every cause of death was on the increase. There were very few plague cases listed, but plenty of deaths from spotted fever and overeating and childbed fever and stillbirths. Infants were supposedly dying of teething, which was then thought to be a deadly condition.

As the death rolls swelled, the reason became obvious: people were hiding plague deaths. When a searcher—one of the old women paid to briefly examine bodies and record the cause of death—came by, nurses would often cover the body, trying to keep it warm because occasionally buboes would not show themselves until a body cooled. Sometimes the searchers noticed anyway, and they would be offered a bribe to fudge the official records.

Nobody wanted to be associated with a plague victim. Plague houses were boarded up, with healthy family still inside, as a form of quarantine. The door would be painted with a red cross and the words "Lord have mercy upon us." Nobody would be allowed to enter or leave until the residents died, or until forty days had passed.

Parishes took care of the family, on paper anyway, if they were poor. A warden stood guard at the door, passing the family whatever food or provisions they asked for, and the family would receive an allowance to buy those supplies. The flaw in this plan was that the watchman had no consequences if he failed to do his job; the family would starve, but hey, they were going to die anyway.

The nurses didn't want to be associated with a plague family, because they would be shut up in the house too. The neighbors knew it would look bad to have plague cases on their street, since the disease—according to rich Londoners, anyway—was supposed to visit the people who were dirtiest and most immoral. Even the searchers had reason to avoid pronouncing plague deaths; in epidemic times, they would have to live in a lean-to in the churchyard, just like the gravediggers.

IN LONDON

Soon, boarded-up plague houses began appearing. The outskirts of town, where the poorest people lived, were hardest hit, but by the end of the year the plague had made its mark almost everywhere in the city.

King Charles II left town, taking along his family and the rest of the court. Almost half of the city's population fled, mainly wealthy families, as it was expensive to hire a fast carriage to take you as far away as possible. And the flight was often too late. A poem teasing the "Run-Awayes" advised them that after fleeing "you are much worse / Having both Plague of Body and of Purse."

People from the surrounding towns realized that travelers might be carrying plague, and kept an eye out especially for the poorer-looking ones. One group of travelers was attacked with clubs at Hayes, another threatened with muskets at Whetstone. The headmaster of King's School in Westminster put students onto boats to leave the city, judging the waterways to be safer than the roads.

Inside the city, festivals were canceled. Taverns and inns were ordered closed. Even private gatherings brought extra attention from the police in case dissenters were plotting an uprising in the king's absence. The only acceptable place to gather was at churches, where special plague services were regularly held.

As the plague claimed more victims, there were no longer enough nurses or wardens to take care of shut-ins, so families with plague were finally allowed to leave home (although they were told to do so at night).

So many bodies piled up in the dead-carts that the city bought suburban land for mass graves, and churches that had space in their yards made money by offering to bury the dead from smaller parishes. Individual graves and coffins became a thing of the past for many folks. In some paupers' burials, each body was dumped into a common pit grave and the coffin reused.

By the fall, the numbers of deaths started to decrease: from 1,400 per week in early November to 210 a month later. The worst was over.

FIRE AND SOAP

This was London's last case of plague. The periodic epidemics stopped after 1665. London's Great Fire sometimes gets the credit, but another likely hero is the growing trend toward cleanliness.

Plague has many ways to travel. In an infected body, the bacteria can fill the bloodstream and wait for a bite from a flea, or if the germs have colonized the lungs, they can make the victim cough blood. This transmission by coughing is known as pneumonic plague, and it's almost 100 percent fatal. Fortunately, plague prefers to travel by flea.

Rat fleas were responsible for bringing plague through Europe in the first place, but they probably can't take the blame for the way plague can fell all the members of a household. Wendy Orent writes in her book *Plague* that the rat flea "moves the disease along, slowly and irregularly, but [the human fleas] cause sudden intense and murderous explosions within households." Those human fleas, *Pulex irritans*, enjoy biting humans but live in clothes and bedding.

Fleas, at the time, were an annoying but unremarkable fact of life, like spiders or fruit flies are in our houses today. But when people got better about keeping clean, fleas became more rare. Plague went back to occasional outbreaks, the same as in the United States today, where a handful of people will contract plague each year but epidemics don't result.

Soap may have taken a while to catch on as a trend, but the Great Fire of 1666 acted more quickly. Before the fire, many of London's roofs were thatch, meaning they were made of straw. Flea-ridden rats could live in thatch roofs, but after the fire, roofs were rebuilt with less flammable materials. Millions of fleas would have perished in bedding, too. The fire might not have made London plague-proof, but it was a good start.

CHAPTER 23

SCOURGE OF A YOUNG NATION'S CAPITAL

YELLOW FEVER: PHILADELPHIA
1793

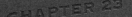

YELLOW FEVER'S INTERNAL BLEEDING AND BLACK VOMIT WERE ENOUGH TO GRIND THE GOVERNMENT TO A HALT, AS POLITICIANS AND PEOPLE FLED FROM THE CITY IN DROVES.

DEATH TOLL: 4,000–5,000 (estimated)

CAUSED BY: Yellow fever virus

NOTEWORTHY SYMPTOMS: Fever, jaundice, black vomit

FATALITY RATE: 20–50 percent in severe cases

THREAT LEVEL TODAY: Low. A vaccine exists, and mosquito control measures keep the disease's spread in check.

NOTABLE FACT: Celebrity first lady Dolley Madison married future president James Madison a year after she was widowed in the yellow fever epidemic.

George Washington was not the first to flee from Philadelphia that year, and he would not be the last. Half the population left the city as an epidemic of yellow fever spread that muggy summer, claiming dozens of victims each day.

Alexander Hamilton was nearly one of them. He fell ill, followed by his wife, Eliza, and they sent their children to stay with family near Albany, New York, while they recovered at home. When they traveled to reunite with the children, they hit literal roadblocks. Cities and towns placed guards on the road to turn away travelers from Philadelphia. The Hamiltons were only allowed to cross the river into Albany by leaving their carriages, servants, and clothing behind.

George Washington sparked a constitutional crisis when he left town expecting the outbreak to be short-lived. Since other government representatives had left the area, and the epidemic raged for months, a regular meeting of Congress was impossible. Hamilton recommended that Congress just meet in another city. But the constitution specifically included a rule that Congress could never meet elsewhere, since English kings were known to suddenly move Parliament to remote locations when they needed to rig a vote. The federal government ground to a halt.

TREATING YELLOW FEVER

Almost nobody guessed where the disease came from, but one anonymous person wrote in to *Dunlap's American Daily Advertiser* with what we now know was the correct answer. The city was full of rain barrels, he (or she) said, teeming with millions of young mosquitoes not quite mature enough to fly away. The writer suggested pouring a few ounces of oil into each barrel to suffocate the mosquitoes. If residents had heeded this advice, the yellow fever virus would have been left without a way to fly around the city.

But that advice was lost amongst all the other recommendations for how to avoid yellow fever. Floors should be covered in fresh dirt, wrote one physician, and changed out every day. People sprinkled vinegar in their houses and breathed through vinegar-soaked handkerchiefs when they went outside. Tobacco smoke, garlic, and bitter-smelling camphor were also thought to be protective. A commission of doctors recommended that the city clean up the streets and burn gunpowder to purify the air.

Here's how a typical course of yellow fever presents itself. In the first few days, a fever appears, accompanied by nausea and headache. The patient then seems to get better, and in most cases the worst is over. But for an unlucky 15 percent or so, the fever returns, this time accompanied by severe pain and by internal bleeding that results in black vomit with clotted blood. The heart and kidneys may fail, but it's the liver damage that gives the disease its name. With the liver out of commission, a blood chemical called bilirubin builds up in the body, turning the patient's skin and eyes a yellowish color. When the disease reaches this stage, as many as half of the patients may die.

Doctors of the city argued bitterly over the right way to treat a patient who was sick with yellow fever. Even today, we don't have a satisfying answer to that question. Yellow fever is caused by a virus, so not even antibiotics can make a sick person better. The modern treatment is to help the patient get rest and fluids, and to provide pain relief and fever reducers as needed.

Alexander Hamilton, once he was recovered, wrote to the College of Physicians of Philadelphia to recommend the approach used by his doctor and friend, Edward Stevens. Dr. Stevens's treatment was gently supportive, involving cold baths, glasses of brandy, and quinine enemas.

Meanwhile, doctors like Benjamin Rush preferred a drastic approach. Since patients vomit up clotted blood, the theory went, the sooner they got rid of that blood the sooner they could recover. Rush had always been a fan of mild bloodletting, a common treatment at the time. But when patients still died in spite of gentle cures, he stepped up his efforts. Patients might be bled until they fainted. They would also receive his "ten and ten" cure: ten grains of a toxic mercury compound, and ten of a powdered poisonous root called jalap. The poisoning resulted in vomiting and diarrhea.

Patients still died, so Dr. Rush increased the dosage. The deaths didn't stop, but at least Dr. Rush, and the doctors who agreed with him, knew that they had tried the most powerful treatments in their toolbox. This approach was known as "heroic" medicine, and it probably sent some of the yellow fever patients to an early grave.

THE CITY RECOVERS

While at first the city was full of panic and rapidly emptying of its citizens, soon the sick were in the care of a few brave souls who stayed and helped their neighbors. The only organized effort, at first, came from the Free African Society. Philadelphia's 40,000 citizens included 200 slaves and 3,000 free blacks. Because of a rumor that African Americans were not susceptible to yellow fever, Dr. Rush wrote to the society to ask for its help. Later, he taught the society's volunteer nurses (who included both men and women) how to bleed patients and administer his favorite treatments.

The nurses witnessed some of the city's saddest scenes. One time, the nurses found a small child in the house where they were sent to pick up a body. She told them "Mamma is asleep, don't wake her." Then she asked why they were putting her mamma in a box. "We did not know how to answer her," they wrote, "but committed her to the care of a neighbor, and left her with heavy hearts."

The volunteer nurses from the Free African Society visited as many sick residents as they could, and were among the few people willing to handle and bury the corpses. Families of the afflicted offered payment, and soon began offering more and more money to secure the services of the overworked nurses. Soon, people were accusing the Free African Society of extortion. Philadelphia's mayor, one of the few government officials who did not leave the city during the outbreak, published a letter applauding the society's work and asking citizens to please not harass the nurses as they went about their jobs.

After the epidemic, leaders of the Free African Society published a pamphlet refuting some of the nastier rumors, pointing out that blacks in fact died at the same rate as whites, and often seemed to catch the disease while caring for white patients. Yet they persevered. "A white man threatened to shoot us if we passed by his house with a corpse," the authors wrote. "We buried him three days later."

Eventually winter came, and the mosquitoes died. Cases of yellow fever dwindled to the single digits, and people returned to the city. The government passed a law to allow Congress to relocate in case of emergency. And the city too moved on, with heavy hearts.

CHAPTER 24

PEEING RED

WHILE FIGHTING IN EGYPT, NAPOLEON'S SOLDIERS CONTRACTED A WORM PARASITE THAT CAUSED THICK, BLOODY, AND PAINFUL URINE THAT THEY HAD TO SUFFER THROUGH FOR THE REMAINDER OF THEIR LIVES—AS IF FIGHTING FOR NAPOLEON WASN'T BAD ENOUGH!

DEATH TOLL: Unknown

CAUSED BY: A tiny worm called *Schistosoma haematobium*

NOTEWORTHY SYMPTOMS: Blood in the urine

FATALITY RATE: Unknown

THREAT LEVEL TODAY: This condition still affects 240 million people worldwide.

NOTABLE FACT: While many of the worm's eggs are peed out, some may become misdirected and clog up the host's organs.

C amping with thousands of fellow soldiers in a faraway land is a reliable prescription for disease. Napoleon Bonaparte's campaign in Egypt, with 38,000 men, was no exception.

Alongside those men came about 300 women: nurses. The general knew that disease follows war, and calculated that one in ten soldiers would get sick, and one in every twenty-five would become wounded. He ordered the army's paymaster to hire as many doctors and surgeons as he could find, and "eight or ten good hospital directors." And still, the men got sick. They got malaria, and the doctors gave them quinine. They got dysentery, and the doctors kept them hydrated. They got syphilis and gonorrhea, and the general ordered the massacre of 400 sex workers.

Bubonic plague was one of the many illnesses that struck the men, and Napoleon himself visited the plague hospital, helping to move a fresh corpse to show he didn't fear the disease. The doctors inoculated themselves with pus from patients' infected lymph nodes to demonstrate to the men that the disease was not contagious. They were wrong, of course. It would be another hundred years before scientists could show that the lymph nodes were teeming with infectious bacteria. Many of the daredevil doctors died.

But there was another disease. In danger of being lost amongst all the plague and dysentery was a poorly understood syndrome that cropped up among the soldiers: they began urinating blood. One of the doctors reported afterward that it was a stubborn disease; he had no cures for it besides fluids and rest. The urine is thick and bloody, he wrote, with pain in the bladder. And even after the men returned home, they found no relief, and faced the sad prospect of suffering from the disease for the rest of their lives.

A PUZZLE

To the doctors, this bloody urine disease was more baffling than plague. An army surgeon named A.J. Renoult blamed the climate: apparently the heat and dryness were harmful to people who weren't used to it. Another doctor, writing later about a similar condition on the island of Mauritius, said that the reason so many children had bloody urine—three-quarters of them—was because of too much spicy food and masturbation.

Skip forward half a century. Theodor Bilharz, a physician in Cairo, was doing an autopsy when he found an unusual type of worm in the veins near the liver. "A look in the microscope revealed a magnificent Distomum with flat body and a twisted tail," he wrote to his mentor Carl von Siebold back home, who later published the letters. "These are a few leaves of a saga as wonderful as the best of the thousand and one nights—if I succeed in putting it all together." People began calling the disease Bilharzia.

The magnificent worm was a male, and soon Bilharz had also found a female. The two spend their adult lives locked together, the female inside the male's wider, grooved body. Imagine a hot dog nestled in a bun. Now imagine that hot dog is hair-thin and half an inch long, and lays eggs in your bladder.

The eggs, each adorned with a single spike, were obviously meant to exit the bladder by urination. But what happened next? How would the worms get back into a human?

Japanese scientists figured out the next page of the story. While a scientist named Matsuura was wading in rice paddies to study a mysterious parasitic disease in the Katayama region of Japan, he was careful to only eat food that had been boiled, just in case a parasite had made its way onto his food or in his drinking water. (Many parasites are transmitted this way.) He came down with the disease he was studying anyway, and later experiments confirmed that you don't have to drink this type of parasite; standing in infected water is all it takes.

SNAIL FEVER

Here's what happens. When a person releases the eggs into a pond or puddle, the eggs hatch and the larvae search for snails. The newborn parasite must burrow into a snail's soft foot in its first twenty-four hours of life, or it becomes just another dead worm on the pond bottom.

Inside the snail, the parasite matures. A new type of worm swims forth, one with a forked tail. This one seeks out human flesh, looks for a breach in the skin—a hair follicle is good enough—and unnoticeably chews its way in.

The person may notice some itchiness where the worm entered. She may brush it off as "just swimmer's itch." But inside, the young worms are already transforming. They find their way to the veins near the bladder (or in other species, like the one in Japan, veins near the rectum). Here, they lay their eggs, and the cycle can begin again.

It's only a new beginning for the worm, though. The person who became their home could be saddled with the worm for life. She is now peeing blood, and may also end up with wayward worm eggs clogging delicate organs. Napoleon himself may have contracted the disease and carried these worms, called *Schistosoma* or sometimes just the blood fluke or snail fluke, throughout his life.

If so, he was just one tiny data point in a long history of *Schistosoma* infections in Egypt. Urologists like to say that the infection appears in ancient Egyptian medical texts, along with suggested remedies, but that's probably a mistranslation; the hieroglyphic word they point to, which includes a picture of a penis, probably refers to an evil spirit instead. If that's true, there is no mention of bloody urine in the medical texts at all, which is remarkable in itself because it would mean the disease may have been so common that nobody went to the doctor about it.

The disease was definitely present in Egypt in ancient times; 3,000-year-old mummies have been found with snail flukes in their body. The snails in question enjoy sunny, stagnant water, and even today they tend to crop up where people build dams or flood rice paddies. In Egypt, the Nile flooded every spring, and farmers used this water to irrigate their crops. Snails and *Schistosoma* would have thrived then just as they do now.

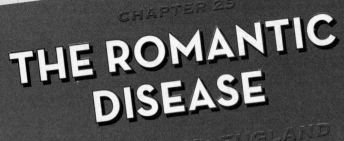

THE ROMANTIC DISEASE

TUBERCULOSIS: ENGLAND
1800s

GROWING PALE AND WASTING AWAY IN THE PRIME OF LIFE: WHAT COULD BE MORE DRAMATIC?

DEATH TOLL: As many as a quarter of all deaths in England in some years

CAUSED BY: The bacterium *Mycobacterium tuberculosis*

NOTEWORTHY SYMPTOMS: Coughing blood, paleness, and weight loss

FATALITY RATE: Nearly 100 percent if untreated (and if you don't die of something else first)

THREAT LEVEL TODAY: 1.3 million people still die of tuberculosis every year. Antibiotic treatments help in many cases.

NOTABLE FACT: Anti-spitting campaigns in the late nineteenth century helped to get tuberculosis-infested spit off the streets.

The nineteenth century had a lot of awful ways to die. By comparison, consumption was almost glamorous.

One Romantic-era heroine after another died a tragic, youthful death, her frail body wasting away while her mind stayed bright, until one day she coughed blood for the last time, and died. These were the fictional stars of *La Bohème* and *La Traviata* and *Les Misérables.* Emily Brontë described the heroine of *Wuthering Heights* as "rather thin, but young and fresh complexioned and her eyes sparkled like diamonds." Edgar Allan Poe made a whole genre out of lamenting the deaths of young women with all the outward signs of the disease: waifish, ghostly pale, angelic.

Consumption may not have been fun, but it sure beat dying of cholera, or smallpox, or one of the epidemics that signaled the last gasps of the Black Death. Consumption was nicknamed the "white plague."

It was common, too. Consumption claimed the lives of many of the same poets and painters who glamorized the disease. It killed all three literary Brontë sisters, plus their other siblings. Poe's very young wife died of the disease, and Poe himself may have had it too. The list goes on and on: Elizabeth Barrett Browning, Henry David Thoreau, Keats, Shelley, Byron, and more. But while consumption provided a tragic end to these illustrious lives, it also slaughtered the poor and working class, children included. Millions perished without a single sonnet to their name.

BUT IS IT CONTAGIOUS?

What the Romantics called "consumption" we would mostly recognize as tuberculosis. The victim would often be somebody who was sickly or weak to begin with, and then a dry cough would develop as the disease ravaged the lungs.

We know now that the disease is caused by bacteria that settle in the lungs and cause pockets of infection. A healthy immune system can usually contain the disease in tiny nodules, which were described at autopsy as "tubercles." They have a cheese-like consistency on the inside, and in somebody with a less than stellar immune system, the bacteria often break out of their tiny cages to cause the bleeding—which was coughed delicately onto a handkerchief, perhaps. The germs can also travel through the bloodstream to create tubercles on other body parts. On lymph nodes in the neck, they create scrofula. They can also settle on bones and organs, causing further disease.

For centuries, experts debated what sort of disease consumption was. One school of thought held that the disease was hereditary, because "consumptives" clustered in families (like the Brontës). On the other hand, maybe it was infectious. But the bacteria that cause tuberculosis grow so slowly that doctors and scientists of the time weren't able to catch the connection.

"If contagion had anything really to do with it, why did it prove so long in showing itself?" wrote physician Henry Bowditch, debating with himself in an 1864 paper titled "Is Consumption Ever Contagious?" While the immune system is fighting the bacteria, or while it has them temporarily contained, months or years may elapse. This made the connection hard to see.

Different theories took hold in different parts of Europe. English physicians saw consumption as a common disease that almost everyone was exposed to (if it was a matter of exposure) and only some people got sick. They focused on why some groups of people got it more than others: women versus men, poor versus wealthy. The situation was reversed in Italy, where consumptives who visited for the healthy sea air could find themselves thrown out of hotels and boardinghouses by people who wanted nothing to do with disease.

Since it wasn't seen as contagious in many places, the blood-flecked phlegm of a person with tuberculosis could safely (they thought) be hocked into the streets. Before contagion was understood, spitting was just an ordinary part of life. Samuel Pepys wrote in 1661 that "a lady spit backward upon me by a mistake [at the theater], not seeing me, but after seeing her to be a very pretty lady, I was not troubled at it at all."

Or as physician C. Theodore Williams wrote in 1882, just after the tuberculosis germ, or bacillus, was discovered: "When we consider the number of consumptive people who, being under no restriction, go about coughing and expectorating freely in the streets and parks of London, we must admit that the bacilli, though ever present, are not very active in ill-doing."

He was right, in a sense. Since so many people could be infected without coming down with obvious symptoms of the disease, infectious spittle was not doing everyone harm. But all cases of tuberculosis resulted from infection. Dr. Robert Koch confirmed this theory in a thorough lecture and demonstration at the University of Berlin's Physiology Institute. He had isolated the germ and proved it was the culprit by infecting hundreds of guinea pigs. That bacterium was known for a time as the "tubercle bacillus," giving the disease its still-current nickname: TB.

THE REMEDY

But knowledge did not lead to a cure. Koch claimed to have one, a mysterious remedy whose ingredients he would not divulge. But it failed as a cure, and in fact reactivated tuberculous lesions that had lain dormant for years. We still use a version of his remedy today, called tuberculin, but not as a treatment. Instead, injecting a drop of it underneath the skin effectively tests whether someone has had the disease.

Even today, our tools for dealing with tuberculosis are not perfect. A vaccine exists, but is only partially effective. (It's not in routine use in the United States.) Antibiotics can kill the germs, but *Mycobacterium tuberculosis* is getting smarter, and some strains are drug-resistant. Today, the disease is mostly kept at bay by preventing its spread.

Back in the Romantic era, conditions in cities helped tuberculosis spread. Factory workers and other poor folks worked long hours on little food, and lived crowded together in tiny, often windowless rooms. *M. tuberculosis* found cities a perfect playground.

The bacterium travels from person to person by droplets in the air, released with a cough or a sneeze. For a while, experts couldn't agree on whether fresh air would make the disease better or worse, so in many cases a family member would care for their loved one in small sooty rooms, afraid to open a window.

John Keats caught the disease in this exact way, nursing one of his brothers, who died of the disease. Years earlier, he had done the same for his mother. He traveled by sea to the supposedly better air of the Mediterranean, sharing a cabin with a young woman who also had tuberculosis. They couldn't agree on whether the porthole should be open or closed. When it was open, he coughed; when it was closed, she fainted.

That was another glamorous aspect to tuberculosis: the cure was often a vacation. Both the sea air of the Mediterranean and the mountain air of the Alps were considered to be excellent places to go. Entire resorts sprang up to cater to the consumptive, later expanding to admit patients and hypochondriacs of all types. Today, instead of a vacation, you get a regimen of multiple antibiotics. Less glamorous, but more effective.

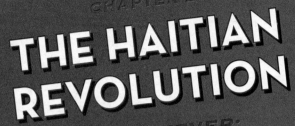

CHAPTER 26

THE HAITIAN REVOLUTION

YELLOW FEVER:
SAINT-DOMINGUE (NOW HAITI)

1802

HAITIAN REBEL SOLDIERS FOUGHT BRAVELY—BUT IT WAS THE DEVASTATING SYMPTOMS OF YELLOW FEVER THAT TIPPED THE BALANCE TO THEIR SIDE.

DEATH TOLL: At least 29,000

CAUSED BY: Yellow fever virus

NOTEWORTHY SYMPTOMS: Fever, jaundice, black vomit

FATALITY RATE: 20–50 percent in severe cases

THREAT LEVEL TODAY: Low in the United States. A vaccine exists, and mosquito control measures keep the disease's spread in check. There are still 200,000 cases each year, with 90 percent in Africa.

NOTABLE FACT: Yellow fever helped to win the first and only successful slave rebellion on record.

Yellow fever probably arrived in Haiti when the slaves did. The first known epidemics date from 1647. Yellow fever and malaria come from Africa, and so does the mosquito that can carry those diseases.

Haiti, then a French colony known as Saint-Domingue, was populated almost entirely by slaves in the 1790s. Only 10 percent of its population were free; the rest worked on plantations, mainly planting and cutting sugar cane and working in the mills and boiling houses. The slaves were so abused and overworked that deaths outpaced births, requiring a steady supply of fresh workers from Africa.

These new arrivals were often former soldiers, captured in civil wars. They had experience fighting and strategizing. As Laurent Dubois writes in *Haiti: The Aftershocks of History*: "All they needed were weapons and opportunity."

That opportunity began with the French Revolution, which inspired both slaves and free people of color to fight for more rights under the law. In 1794, the French outlawed slavery in all of their colonies. A new system emerged on Saint-Domingue, where the former slaves became "cultivators" who were still tied to their land, but now received a 25 percent share of the plantation's profits. They were also able to expand the plots of land on which they grew food and raised livestock. One former slave owner, returning after the uprising, asked the workers on his plantation for some food. There are potatoes in the garden, he was told. Help yourself.

At this point, Saint-Domingue was still a French colony, and the rebellion's leader, Toussaint L'Ouverture, was its governor. But when Napoleon Bonaparte took over the French government, with the help of his brother-in-law Charles Leclerc, he looked across the ocean and saw the situation in Saint-Domingue unacceptable. He sent Leclerc by sea with a small army, saying their purpose was to keep the peace, but privately told Leclerc to "rid us of these gilded negroes."

TINY ALLIES

Half of the island's former slaves had been born in Africa, and had recently stepped off the slave ships, sometimes with fresh brands burned onto their chests, with mosquitoes buzzing around their ears. Barrels of drinking water, carried on the ships, were the perfect nursery for baby mosquitoes. Several generations of the insects lived and died in the time it took to sail the Atlantic.

The mosquito that carries yellow fever is known to scientists as *Aedes aegypti*. It can also carry other viruses, including dengue, chikungunya, and Zika. Both males and females drink nectar from flowers, but the female needs extra protein when it's time to lay eggs. That's when she goes looking for a blood meal.

Most of the time *Aedes aegypti* is a slim dark-colored mosquito with white spots on its abdomen and legs. When the female drinks blood, the meal expands the mosquito's thin body, turning it plump and stretching it so the red shows through. After she has digested the blood, she lays 100 to 200 eggs on a damp surface that's likely to flood. In rainforests, that might be a hole in a tree. On a ship, or in a city, the mosquito can breed in rain barrels, tin cans, swamps, or anywhere the water is still. They will hatch in two days if they stay wet and the weather is warm; they can survive for two months if they dry out.

If the mother mosquito bites someone who has yellow fever, she takes up the virus along with the blood. The virus replicates inside her gut, and migrates through her body to her salivary glands. She'll inject that saliva into her next victim, because mosquitoes' saliva contains chemicals that keep blood from clotting. In doing so, she will pass on the virus. The female *Ae. aegypti* needs a new blood meal for each batch of eggs, so over her lifetime she may have several opportunities to spread disease. The virus can also spread inside of her, colonizing her ovaries so that when she lays eggs, the young are already infected.

These mosquitoes found homes in containers and puddles and ponds on the plantations and in the port cities of Saint-Domingue.

They didn't bother many of the new arrivals, who had already come down with yellow fever back home, perhaps in childhood. But for the Europeans, the new disease was much more likely to strike, and to be deadly.

THE MOSQUITOES WIN

Leclerc and his troops arrived in 1802, and were astounded to find that both sides of the war were singing the same French revolutionary anthems, fighting for different variations of the same cause. One rebel general had ripped out the white stripe of the French flag to create a red-and-blue banner for a nation he hoped would no longer be run by whites.

Toussaint L'Ouverture knew he could not hold the port cities, so he ordered them burned to the ground. He then led the French troops into the interior of the island, where he hoped he would only have to outlast them through the yellow fever season. L'Ouverture was captured, and he died in a remote French prison, but his strategy eventually worked. The French soldiers numbered 29,000 when they arrived, and proceeded to kill 150,000 Haitians, nearly a third of the population. But the French fared proportionately worse: thanks partly to combat deaths but largely to yellow fever, 26,000 French soldiers died. Their general, Leclerc, was one of the casualties.

Haiti was forced to pay France in 1825 for the slave owners' property losses, even though slavery had already been outlawed. The payment sent Haiti into a spiral of poverty that continues today. And France, unable to win a war in *Aedes aegypti* territory, withdrew from the area. A year later, it sold the Louisiana territory to the United States, changing the course of that nation's history, too.

CHAPTER 27

BIRTH OF A PANDEMIC

CHOLERA: INDIA
1817

THE MOST FAMOUS OF THE WORLD'S DIARRHEAL DISEASES LEAVES ITS BIRTHPLACE AND TAKES A DEADLY TOUR AROUND THE WORLD.

DEATH TOLL: Unknown, but very large

CAUSED BY: The bacterium *Vibrio cholerae*

NOTEWORTHY SYMPTOMS: Extreme diarrhea that kills by dehydration

FATALITY RATE: More than 50 percent without treatment

THREAT LEVEL TODAY: Low in high-income countries; high in areas without reliable sewers and clean water.

NOTABLE FACT: The *Vibrio* bacteria that causes food poisoning from oysters is a close relative of cholera.

The Ganges River begins with melting snow from the Himalayan Mountains, and it winds 1,500 miles east through the tropical climate of northern India as its tributaries combine to form the river that the Hindu religion considers the sacred territory of the goddess Ganga. Bathing in the river, and drinking from it, transform an ordinary routine into a religious experience. People from all over India travel to the Ganges, following wide steps down into the river. A bottle of the water, taken home, is part souvenir and part holy relic.

The river crosses into neighboring Bangladesh and ends at the Bay of Bengal, flowing into the Indian Ocean. The city of Kolkata is not far away. It is here, in the Bengal region, that cholera may have first learned to infect people, giving them such terrible diarrhea that they die of dehydration. That diarrhea, in turn, can infect many others if it makes its way to a water source—either a pond or well, or perhaps even the Ganges itself.

The first recorded pandemic of cholera traces back to 1817, when it started in the Bengal region—or possibly in Jessore in Bangladesh—and ultimately toured half the world. It was the first of many; so far the world has survived at least seven cholera pandemics, and an eighth may be emerging.

Cholera may have visited other parts of the world before this first recognized pandemic. Hippocrates and other physicians and writers of the Middle East and Europe wrote descriptions of a disease with copious watery diarrhea. They called it cholera, but we don't know if it was a true relation of the fatal disease that traveled out of India in 1817.

Where rivers meet oceans, a special habitat occurs: an estuary, where fresh water and salt water mix. This is where bacteria in the genus *Vibrio* are happiest. Some members of that family infect shellfish, and are a source of seafood-related food poisoning. *Vibrio cholerae* started this way, attaching itself to plants and plankton in the warm water. It lived in or on shellfish and insects, probably not causing much trouble—until it discovered how to infect people.

Vibrio cholerae's DNA looks similar to its less harmful relatives, except for a few genes that spell disaster for humans who come too close. One contains the instructions to make a toxin, called simply "cholera toxin"; other genes provide the equipment to control when that toxin will be produced and to feed it to nearby human cells.

When a person swallows *Vibrio cholera*—perhaps in a gulp of contaminated water—some of the bacteria are killed by stomach acids, but a few may make it to the intestines, where the cholera toxin does its work. Normally, one of the intestines' jobs is to make sure not too much precious water gets excreted. That's why, even though the stomach mixes food with copious squirts of gastric juice, the feces that leave the body are mostly solid. The extra liquid has all been reabsorbed. If the body were not so careful about conserving water, we would quickly dehydrate.

The cholera toxin throws a wrench in this process, in effect reversing it—turning on the tap and letting it run. Water flows out of the bowels, first as diarrhea, then simply as a thin milky liquid. Within hours, a person can become so dehydrated that she dies.

But the bacterium is not the only one with special genes that ensure its survival. Recent DNA studies have shown that the people whose families lived in the Bengal region for generation upon generation have genes that protect them from cholera. They are less likely to get sick, thanks to their specialized immune response, which helps but isn't perfect protection. These protective powers also explain why the people in that area need larger doses of cholera vaccine than people from other parts of the world do: their immune systems don't get excited about just any cholera germ that floats by.

GOING FOR A RIDE

In 1817, cholera was a familiar disease to the Indians who lived in the germ's regular stomping grounds. It did kill people, and it did spread in occasional epidemics, from Bengal to southern India, for example, or sometimes in the opposite direction. What spurred the disease to spread so suddenly is not clear, but British invasion probably had something to do with it. First the disease appeared in the northeast corner of the country and began spreading locally. Then it went farther across India, possibly aided by one of the Kumbh Mela festivals that brought hundreds of thousands, even millions of people to the banks of the Ganges for communal prayer and bathing. From this pilgrimage, travelers could have taken the disease to the rest of the country.

From there, thanks to military and cargo ships, it spread far and fast. By 1818 it was in Bombay (now Mumbai) and Ceylon (Sri Lanka). To the east, it hit Burma (Myanmar) in 1819, then Thailand, Penang, and Singapore by 1820. By the time it entered Beijing by sea in 1820, it had already been in southern China for three years thanks to the shorter travel by land. In 1822, a ship brought it from Java to Japan.

Neither British nor Indian physicians had any good ideas about how to treat or stop cholera. (Even today, our best treatment is to simply keep the person hydrated until the disease runs its course.) The British were still working from a theory about needing to balance the four humors, and their main medical tools were bloodletting and drugs that would cause vomiting and even more diarrhea. Indians weren't as big on bloodletting, but otherwise their approach was similar, based on an idea about three humors that needed to be balanced: air, bile, and phlegm. Neither approach explained, or stopped, the rampage of *Vibrio cholerae.*

The disease spread west, too. In 1821, a battle in Oman, near the southeast corner of Saudi Arabia, involved British soldiers that had been in India. The disease spread from there, into modern-day Iran, Syria, Iraq, and parts of Russia. Eventually it fizzled out, perhaps stopped or slowed by a cold winter in 1824.

But the world would not be so lucky for long. A few years later, in 1827, a new pandemic started, at first tracing the westward steps of the first one. From the Middle East, a branch infected parts of Africa. Another branch proceeded through Russia to western Europe and from there to the Americas. This was not the last we would see of cholera.

CHAPTER 28

CHILDBED FEVER

UTERINE INFECTION: VIENNA
1847

WOMEN WERE DYING IN DROVES FROM INFECTIONS AFTER CHILDBIRTH. THE DRASTIC AND SIMPLE SOLUTION: TELLING DOCTORS TO WASH THEIR HANDS.

DEATH TOLL: Up to 500 per year

CAUSED BY: A variety of bacteria, including Group A *Streptococcus*

NOTEWORTHY SYMPTOMS: Swollen, painful uterus; fever; foul-smelling vaginal discharge

FATALITY RATE: 80–90 percent in risky settings

THREAT LEVEL TODAY: Medium. The potential for infection still exists, but it's kept at bay with measures that include hand washing and antibiotics.

NOTABLE FACT: Researchers estimate that if everybody washed their hands, including outside of hospital settings by washing after using the bathroom and before eating, 1 million deaths per year (mostly from diarrheal disease) could be prevented.

G iving birth is one of the most dangerous things a woman can do. It was even more dangerous in the 1800s, and disastrously so at certain hospitals. The Allgemeines Krankenhaus in Vienna, Austria, was just one of many where 20 percent of new mothers were dead within ten days.

But that number only applied to half of the hospital: the First Division, where doctors and medical students delivered the babies. Just across the hall in the Second Division, where births were attended by students and teachers of midwifery, death rates were minuscule.

Ignaz Semmelweis, newly appointed assistant to the director of the First Division, noticed the difference. Everybody did, since the hospital kept careful records, but nobody had found a way to change the mortality rates.

The women were dying of what was then called puerperal fever. Today we would recognize it as a massive bacterial infection starting in the uterus. Hundreds of years ago, doctors hadn't heard of germs; fevers were thought to come from breathing foul air, or bad mixes of humors in the body.

During the eighteenth and nineteenth centuries, autopsies became a popular way to sharpen medical knowledge. Upon opening up a woman who had died of puerperal fever, the doctors and students at Allgemeines Krankenhaus would have noticed that the uterus was swollen and inflamed, with pockets of pus either centered on the reproductive organs or dotted around the body. The white blobs of pus gave rise to one of the theories about puerperal fever: since the doctors thought milk comes from blood that has been diverted from the uterus to the breast (it doesn't, of course), the milk must have been blocked somehow, and the white blobs were clotted milk.

Another theory was inspired by the fluid inside the swollen uterus. Since a fluid called lochia normally flows from the uterus after birth—women experience this as bleeding like a heavy period—puerperal fever must mean the flow of lochia was blocked.

But neither of these theories could explain why two otherwise identical groups of patients had such different mortality rates. So after autopsying puerperal fever victims—there were about two deaths every day—the doctors would shrug, wipe the blood off their hands, and head up to the maternity ward to deliver more babies.

DIRTY HANDS

The doctors and students on the ward were fond of doing frequent vaginal examinations on women in labor. This is still done today. Any time you hear a birth story in which somebody tells you how many centimeters dilated they were, that information came from a doctor's or midwife's fingers. Years before Semmelweis, the director of the department was a man who subscribed to a more gentle school of thought. Exams should be kept to a minimum, he decreed, and tools like forceps only used as a last resort. He also only used dead women's bodies for quick autopsies, not as hands-on teaching models. This had a happy side effect: death rates under his direction were as low as the midwife division. And years before that, several doctors had published their theories that maybe, just maybe, doctors and midwives carried childbed fever from one home birth to another. If someone had a string of patients die, he or she might take a bath and change their clothes. One doctor was reported to shave his head and buy a new set of boots, all in vain.

Semmelweis was not the first to suggest that puerperal fever was carried by doctors, but he was the first to do something about it. When a colleague of his died, Semmelweis made a critical connection. The doctor had been cut by a student's knife during an autopsy, and days later died with all the same symptoms of sepsis as the women in the ward. If something from the cadaver had infected the doctor, Semmelweis later wrote, wasn't it possible that "cadaver particles" were infecting women too?

Semmelweis put a bowl of water containing chloride of lime at the entrance to the maternity ward. He didn't know that chloride killed bacteria, since bacteria weren't yet known as a source of disease. He knew just that it tended to neutralize the stench of death that was otherwise detectable on doctors' hands.

Semmelweis ordered all staff and students to wash their hands (and use the provided nail brushes) before attending any of the patients. Infection rates plummeted. The following year, both divisions of the hospital recorded death rates just over 1 percent.

This new idea was controversial. Semmelweis had supporters who argued for its logic, and detractors who couldn't figure out what "cadaver particles" were supposed to be, or whether they even existed. Semmelweis never thought to use the then-new gadget, the microscope, to investigate.

A HARD MESSAGE TO HEAR

No doctor wants to hear that their routine way of working was responsible for the deaths of thousands of patients. Semmelweis was appalled at the realization that he and his colleagues had killed their patients, and worked to change how things were done. Other doctors reacted with denial. It didn't help that Semmelweis called them murderers.

Even after the hand-washing rule was instituted, small outbreaks still occurred. But Semmelweis tracked them down. In one case, a woman on the ward had breast cancer with an ulcer that leaked pus. In another, a woman had a knee infection. Semmelweis amended his theory to say that contamination from any infected person can cause puerperal fever, not just that from cadavers.

Semmelweis instituted similar rules at his next place of employment, but staff tried to sneak by the disinfectant basin without washing their hands, and the hospital administration complained that he spent too much money on bed sheets (since he insisted that they be frequently washed). He delivered a few lectures on his ideas about hand washing, but never wrote a clear, readable paper explaining his position. Ultimately, his detractors were louder.

Hand washing as a medical practice fell by the wayside, not to be resurrected until a surgeon named Joseph Lister read about Louis Pasteur's work on bacteria. He found bacteria in pus he examined under the microscope, experimented with disinfectants, and published the results. The "germ theory" of infection would thus be born—but not until 1867.

CHAPTER 29

MAPPING DEATH

CHOLERA: LONDON
1854

A PARTICULARLY NASTY STRAIN OF CHOLERA RIPS THROUGH LONDON—AND SOME DETECTIVE WORK TRACES IT BACK TO A SINGLE PUMP.

DEATH TOLL: 700 on Broad Street; 10,000 in London that year; over 1,000,000 for the entire third pandemic.

CAUSED BY: The bacterium *Vibrio cholerae*

NOTEWORTHY SYMPTOMS: Diarrhea leading to extreme dehydration

FATALITY RATE: 50 percent or more if untreated

THREAT LEVEL TODAY: Low in high-income countries; high in areas without reliable sewers and clean water.

NOTABLE FACT: John Snow's map of cases is considered a founding moment in the field of epidemiology (the study of diseases and how they spread).

The epidemic began in a slummy Soho neighborhood described as one of the most crowded in London, where human waste piled up in the basements of more than a few houses. Amid this filth, authorities said, it was no surprise that a horrific affliction should begin claiming lives. After all, they said, bad smells are what cause disease.

This disease was cholera, a form of diarrhea so severe it kills more than half of its victims in a matter of days. Cholera outbreaks happened from time to time in nineteenth-century London, but they were never as devastating as this one. In the space of two weeks nearly 700 people died, almost all in a tiny neighborhood centered around Broad Street.

This epidemic would go down in history as the first one in which investigators used data to track down a disease and pinpoint its source: in this case, a contaminated water pump. What makes this feat really amazing is that scientists didn't yet know that germs like bacteria cause disease. The people who solved the mystery, Dr. John Snow and Rev. Henry Whitehead, just knew that there was something about the water in that particular pump. But to make their case, they had to argue against the prevailing theory: that diseases like cholera are caused by breathing in a "miasma" of bad air.

WHERE CHOLERA CAME FROM

Cholera swept over the earth in seven pandemics. The first began around 1817; the seventh started in the 1960s and is still going strong today in some parts of the world. In most of the waves, the pandemic started in India, probably the Bengal region near Kolkata. The bacterium that causes cholera, *Vibrio cholerae*, thrives there as an endemic disease.

From India, the third cholera pandemic spread westward across Asia, hitting the pandemic jackpot at Mecca, where thousands of Muslims visit in an annual pilgrimage. Cholera followed some of the pilgrims to their homes, and soon there were cholera outbreaks across the world. Mexico and Paris were hit hard; forty-niners in

California mining camps also succumbed. Russia lost an estimated 1 million people. The poor of London, living in close quarters with no safe way to dispose of human waste, saw outbreaks every few years.

The *Vibrio cholerae* bacterium is a tiny cell shaped like a curved hot dog with a long whip-like tail at one end. If you ingest *V. cholerae* with about 10 million of its friends, it will feed a protein called cholera toxin to your intestinal cells. The toxin tricks cells into spewing out water nonstop. Victims soon run out of the standard brown liquid we think of as diarrhea, and soon are passing quart after quart of milky white liquid: water containing flaked-off intestinal cells and, as a bonus, trillions of nasty hot dog–shaped bacteria. If these bacteria get onto a caregiver's hands or food, or if they get dumped into the water supply, they can infect another person and the cycle begins again.

The cause of death is dehydration. Those quarts of water leaving the body have been sucked from the bloodstream. With less liquid in the blood, the heart has to beat faster to keep it flowing. Eventually, there isn't enough blood to go around. The patient's kidneys and other organs begin to fail. The brain shifts into unconsciousness or coma, and finally the patient may die.

Doctors in Dr. Snow's time hadn't figured out the simple cure: water. In modern cholera outbreaks, patients are laid on a cot with a hole cut out and a bucket placed underneath it. Nurses check the amount of watery stool in the bucket and make sure the patient gets the same amount of fluid. This low-tech treatment reduces the fatality rate to just 1 percent.

DR. SNOW'S MAP

John Snow had been trying for years to prove that stinky air was not the cause of cholera. He had proposed that water was the culprit, and pointed out that people who die in outbreaks tend to share the same water source. On the other hand, his critics pointed out, those people also live in the same stinky neighborhoods.

The cholera outbreak on Broad Street turned out to be the perfect test for his hypothesis. Dr. Snow looked up the addresses of people who had died, and found that they clustered around the water pump on Broad Street—but there were some anomalies in the data. First, some deaths occurred far away from the pump, and second, inside the outbreak area were some large buildings, a workhouse and a brewery, where almost nobody got sick. These quirks turned out to be the clincher in Dr. Snow's theory.

Dr. Snow went door-to-door in the neighborhood, asking residents where they got their water. One of the faraway cases was a woman who often asked her sons to bring her some water from Broad Street, since she thought it tasted better than the water from her own neighborhood. Other distant cases followed a similar pattern: children who passed the Broad Street pump on their walk home from school often took a swig, and some of these children died in the outbreak. Another of the neighborhood pumps was known for muddy water, so people living near that pump often walked the extra couple of blocks for the famously cool clear water of Broad Street.

There were also people inside the outbreak area who never got sick; for example, all 70 workers at the brewery in the area stayed healthy, and only a few of the 535 occupants of the local workhouse caught the disease. These buildings turned out to have their own water supplies, so the workers and residents never had to drink from the Broad Street pump.

Armed with this evidence, Dr. Snow requested that local officials remove the handle from the Broad Street pump. Cases were already declining—this was a week after the outbreak started, and it was burning out fast—but they agreed to disable the pump. The cholera deaths soon slowed and stopped.

At first, nobody knew why this pump's water should be so toxic. The Board of Health, after removing the pump handle, conducted its own investigation and concluded, again wrongly, that the outbreak was caused by bad air, just as it had thought all along. The reasoning: the well that supplied the Broad Street pump was in proper working order, and the houses where people had died were full of filth and stink—just like every other house in London's overcrowded neighborhoods.

But then Dr. Snow showed his map of the outbreak to Rev. Henry Whitehead, who ministered to the people in the neighborhood, and who at first didn't believe in the bad air theory or the bad water theory. Whitehead questioned more residents, including some who had fled the city as soon as the outbreak started, and he found the source of the outbreak.

The first person to show symptoms of cholera in London in 1854 was a baby girl, who later died. Nobody knows how she contracted cholera, but it turns out the baby's family lived on Broad Street, right next to the pump. Her mother had washed the sick baby's diapers and dumped the water in a cesspit just three feet away from the well. On Whitehead's urging, the cesspit was excavated, and was found to be leaking into the water that supplied the well. The only other time a cholera victim had used the cesspit was the same day the pump's handle was removed, when the baby's father fell ill. If the handle hadn't been removed, a second outbreak might have occurred.

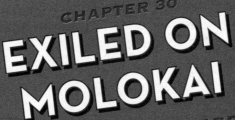

CHAPTER 30
EXILED ON MOLOKAI

LEPROSY (HANSEN'S DISEASE): HAWAII

1866

THOUGHT LEPER COLONIES WERE A THING OF THE PAST? THINK AGAIN. HAWAIIANS WITH LEPROSY WERE IMPRISONED EVEN IN RECENT TIMES.

DEATH TOLL: 8,000 over the years (various causes)

CAUSED BY: The bacterium *Mycobacterium leprae*

NOTEWORTHY SYMPTOMS: Skin lesions, nerve damage

FATALITY RATE: 15 percent on Molokai in the early years, but mainly from infection and not leprosy itself

THREAT LEVEL TODAY: Low. The disease still exists in some countries, but can be treated with antibiotics.

NOTABLE FACT: A few residents still live on Kalaupapa, which has been designated a national park.

M olokai, an island in the world's most isolated archipelago, has one spot that is even more isolated than the rest of it. On its northern coast a volcano once laid out a patch of lava, level with the ocean, at the foot of the sea cliffs. The resulting land reminded somebody of a flat leaf, and that is where it gets its Hawaiian name: Kalaupapa.

Isolation was key to the spot's being chosen as Hawaii's leper colony. In 1866, leprosy was seen as contagious and shameful. Those who had the disease—and probably some people who did not—were sent here. By that time, the native Hawaiian population had already been ravaged by disease. New arrivals of diseases like syphilis, measles, and smallpox were largely responsible for reducing the population from over half a million to an 1850 census count of just 84,000 native Hawaiians.

When leprosy began to appear, the Hawaiians did not know they were supposed to react with disgust. And so the Europeans and Americans who made up the health board were doubly disgusted, both by the people with leprosy and by their families' reaction. In truth, leprosy is not very contagious. Ninety-five percent of people are not susceptible to it, and most people who show symptoms are not in a stage of the infection at which they can pass it to others. But the Europeans were horrified that people with leprosy walked free in the streets instead of hiding in homes or hospitals. Hawaii's King Kamehameha V wanted to stop the deaths of his people from the many diseases that plagued them, and asked the legislature to address the problem. They did: they passed a law criminalizing leprosy.

People with leprosy were to be taken to a hospital near Honolulu for treatment, and those deemed incurable would be taken to Kalaupapa, where houses and farm fields would be waiting for them. They were allowed to bring family members with them to help with chores and provide medical assistance. And so the first group of patients arrived in January 1866. The men were given an axe or shovel and a blanket; the women were just given a blanket.

There had been months of delay in finding a boat and waiting for the seas to calm down enough to get to the island. In the meantime, the crops in the field had rotted. The patients suffered from starvation and infection. Leprosy is not a fatal condition, but in the first five years, 46 percent of the exiles died.

A CURE

Seven years after the colony was founded, Gerhard Hansen peered through a microscope in Norway and saw rod-shaped bacteria in a snippet of skin taken from a patient with leprosy. Neither he nor rival microbiologist Albert Neisser, who first published a description of the germ, could find a way to grow it in the lab. It turned out to be one of the slowest-growing bacteria known, and still has never been grown outside of human or animal cells.

The bacterium, now known as *Mycobacterium leprae*, is a close relative of the one that causes tuberculosis. Scientists attempted to prove it was contagious by conducting human experiments on Kalaupapa, exposing healthy people to fluid from the sores of people with leprosy. Since most people are not susceptible, the experiments often failed. Nineteen years after the colony was founded, in 1885, Hansen's homeland of Norway passed its own law to isolate leprosy patients. This one required the patients to live in hospitals if they did not have their own room at home. The United States dedicated a national leprosarium in 1894 in Carville, Louisiana. It did not close until 1999.

Time passed. Kalaupapa's population swelled to a peak of 1,100 in 1890. Robert Louis Stevenson and Jack London both visited the island and wrote about it. A priest named Father Damien lived in the colony and eventually contracted leprosy himself. After he died, he was canonized. A nun named Mother Marianne took over his job, but never caught the illness. She, too, was canonized after her death.

Seventy-five years after the colony was founded, in 1941, work at Carville resulted in a treatment for leprosy. The drug was a sulfone antibiotic, and was usually taken for life. It could not reverse damage that had already been done to the body, but it could prevent it from progressing any further. A person taking the drug was not contagious. Leprosy became a curable disease.

THE COLONY LIVES ON

Amazingly, the law criminalizing leprosy was not repealed until 1969. The cure had been available for more than twenty-five years; Hawaii had been an American state for a decade. By then, an estimated 8,000 people had been sent to the island, most against their will, torn from their families. Many had leprosy, but some were found to have other, unrelated skin conditions. The island's massive graveyard only has about 1,000 readable stones. A group of former patients and family members is now working to collect residents' names, photographs, and stories. In the 103 years of the colony's existence, thousands of couples had married, and thousands of children had been born. After 1931, babies were taken away from their parents, for fear they would contract leprosy. When the residents of Kalaupapa became free to leave, many did not. The community had become their home, and to leave would be a second uprooting.

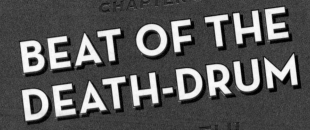

CHAPTER 31

BEAT OF THE DEATH-DRUM

MEASLES: FIJI

1875

THE ROYAL FAMILY OF FIJI HAD NEVER SEEN MEASLES BEFORE—AND NEITHER HAD ANYBODY ELSE IN THE ISLAND NATION. THE RESULTS WERE DEVASTATING.

DEATH TOLL: Estimated at 36,000

CAUSED BY: The measles virus

NOTEWORTHY SYMPTOMS: Fever and a red rash that spreads over the body

FATALITY RATE: About a quarter of the islands' population died

THREAT LEVEL TODAY: Measles still kills over 100,000 people each year. An effective vaccine is available.

NOTABLE FACT: The outbreak could have been prevented if the ships carrying people infected with measles had observed the traditional quarantine protocol of putting up a yellow flag.

When the king of Fiji signed over his islands to the British Empire, he probably envisioned a prosperous future for the new colony. He couldn't have known that an epidemic would sweep through, killing a third of the population in the space of just six months.

The chief, or Ratu, Seru Epenisa Cakobau was the second and last king of Viti, the islands we today call Fiji. His father had declared himself king, although most of the chiefs on the other eighty-some islands didn't recognize him as anything other than an equal. Cakobau inherited the title and waged war against the other chiefs, definitively conquering the islands he felt should be already under his royal power.

This was a tough time to be a ruler of a nation of scattered islands, especially ones that were not so sure they wanted to be a nation. Fiji is in the middle of the Pacific, roughly halfway between Hawaii and Australia. People had been living there since at least 2000 B.C.E., trading via canoes with their neighbors in Polynesian and Micronesian islands. Fijian boats and pottery have been found thousands of miles away from where they were made.

In the 1800s, traders came looking for sandalwood and sea cucumbers; Europeans came to set up plantations of sugar and cotton, staffed by indentured servants. Cakobau thought it would be a good idea to have the British navy on his side, and proposed that Fiji be their newest colony. They turned him down at least once before accepting, in 1874. Papers were signed and the British began to work out the details of the bureaucracy that would run the islands. In the meantime, they invited Cakobau to visit Sydney, Australia.

Cakobau brought his wife, his sons, and a retinue of courtly figures and servants that totaled between 50 and 100 people. They traveled on the HMS *Dido*, and many of the passengers used the docked ship as their hotel, while the people formerly known as the king and queen of Fiji stayed in Sydney itself. They met local dignitaries, and the king was reportedly impressed by magnets and elevators. When the trip was over, they boarded the boat again and set off for home. What nobody realized was that Sydney was in the midst of a minor measles epidemic and that the king's eldest son had, while on shore, taken a good whiff of the virus.

EXPLOSIVELY CONTAGIOUS

Measles isn't just catchy; it's explosively contagious. If nobody in the population is immune, each measles-infected patient will spread the disease to twenty others, on average. The comparable number in AIDS is two to five, and in smallpox, five to seven. Meanwhile, if you haven't had measles (or a measles vaccine) you have a 90 percent chance of contracting the disease if you're exposed to it. In a familiar population, measles can spread quickly from child to child, until everyone is infected and immune—or, in a small percentage of cases, dead. In a fresh population that has never seen the disease before, nearly everyone will catch it.

Tiny clusters of measles virus can hang in the air for hours after somebody with the disease coughs or sneezes. Once the next person breathes in the virus, it incubates in his body for anywhere from one to three weeks. First, the person develops a high fever, perhaps with a runny nose and cough. An observant doctor might note little spots in the mouth that look like grains of salt stuck to the inside of the cheeks. During this stage, the person is already contagious.

Next, a rash breaks out, starting on the face and extending down the body to the arms and legs. It's a flat, red, speckled or blotchy rash. (In older historical records, it's hard to tell if an epidemic was due to measles or smallpox unless the rash is described very specifically. This one was diagnosed by British doctors who, we can be pretty sure, knew measles when they saw it.)

THE EPIDEMIC BEGINS

The king's son Timoci developed a rash when the ship was on its way back home. A chaplain developed it too. The ship's doctor recognized it as measles, and quarantined the men in a small hut on deck to avoid infecting the rest of the people onboard. But that was not all Timoci had picked up. Instead of sleeping peacefully onboard the ship each night, he had been sneaking out and exploring Sydney's brothels. He came down with a case of gonorrhea. When the boat arrived in port, officials onboard were deep in discussions about political damage control, should word of the young man's gonorrhea get out to the press. Timoci was recently married, and the last thing the British officials wanted was a sex scandal.

In the meantime, boats were taking passengers to shore, and the colony's administrator boarded the boat to say hello, accompanied by a good chunk of the police force. These would be the next people to catch measles: all 147 of the men in the police barracks would come down with the disease.

What *should* have happened was that, upon approaching the port, the captain would raise a yellow flag to indicate quarantine. He didn't. The police attempted to spread the news by word of mouth, but officials later reported that the Fijians didn't understand that the disease was serious. They also didn't quarantine two other ships that arrived soon afterward, both from Sydney and with active measles cases onboard.

While the king was on his diplomatic vacation, some of the chiefs from other islands had threatened to revolt, and the king's brother invited them all to meet with the king and other officials when the party returned from the trip. Shortly after the royal family left the boat, then, they were playing host to the new colony's sixty-nine regional chiefs, who along with their attendants made up hundreds of people. After meeting with each other, the chiefs and their retinues got back in their canoes and carried the measles virus to every inhabited island in the archipelago. The devastation was unspeakable. The British later shrugged it off as a culling of an inferior population. The Fijians, meanwhile, thought that the British were poisoning them.

In 1884, a colonial surgeon named Bolton Corney explained the situation to the Epidemiological Society of London. Measles hit every part of Fiji almost simultaneously, and when it did, it wiped out whole villages. There was nobody to fetch water, to harvest or gather food, or to provide any nursing care. The people were terrified, and in some cases ran away from infected houses and refused to have anything to do with their sick loved ones.

Many also refused to take any food or medicine from the British, and steered clear of hospitals. The surgeon reported, appalled, that the Fijians' main strategy to cool the heat of a fever was to lie down in a stream or on wet ground. This, the surgeon said, added to the death toll with pneumonia and dysentery. People also died of dehydration or starvation, in addition to measles, because the loved ones who could otherwise help them were dead, sick, or gone.

He quoted a magistrate who had been away during the few short months of the epidemic. "On my return here, I found death, desolation, and starvation . . . Whole families have been carried off, and, but for the incessant beat of the death-drum, one might fancy the place deserted." By the time the disease completed its tour of the island, the estimated death toll was at least a quarter of the archipelago's total population.

CHAPTER 32

TUNNEL OF ANEMIA

HOOKWORM: SWITZERLAND
1880

Tunnel workers grow pale and weak, and die with worms in their intestines. Turns out it didn't matter that their Swiss water was ultra-clean; this parasite burrowed in through their skin.

DEATH TOLL: Unknown

CAUSED BY: The hookworm *Ancylostoma duodenale*

NOTEWORTHY SYMPTOMS: Weakness, blood loss

FATALITY RATE: Hookworm often contributes to other causes of death rather than killing the victim directly. One estimate in children puts the fatality rate at 7 percent of severe cases.

THREAT LEVEL TODAY: Hookworms affect 740 million people worldwide. Anti-parasitic drugs are available.

NOTABLE FACT: Hookworm infection was common in workplaces where there was no opportunity to use a toilet (like mines and tunnels).

The nine-mile-long St. Gotthard railway tunnel through the Swiss Alps was destined to make history. It would be an important part of international trade, bypassing French railroad monopolies by running through Switzerland instead. It would also be a marvel of engineering, representing the first large-scale use of dynamite for blasting. The tunnel was sure to make the history books. It just had to get built first.

Like other large construction projects of the time, this railway tunnel claimed hundreds of lives in construction. Some workers were killed by the compressed-air trains that carried loads of rock to the outside. Others were killed by sudden floods of water. A few were shot by the Swiss army during an attempted strike. There was another cause of death, too. One that alarmed public health people, especially back in Italy where many of the workers had come from. Workers were staggering out of the tunnel pale and weak, wasting away while their colleagues were, if not healthy, at least healthier.

Some of the Italians headed for home, unable to keep working. One of them, at autopsy, had 1,500 tiny worms attached to the inside walls of his intestines. They were a type that scientists had been studying but didn't yet understand very well, called hookworm. Living miners who displayed symptoms of the wasting disease had hookworm eggs in their feces.

The worms and eggs, by themselves, didn't prove why the miners were getting sick. The worms might not be the cause, argued some of the scientists in the debate that followed. Maybe they got sick for some other reason, and the worms were a minor, irrelevant detail. The worm deniers pointed to the workers' impeccable water source, since parasites typically enter the body through drinking water. Rather than a well subject to contamination, their water came from fresh Alpine streams, brought to the workers by shiny modern steel pipes. The workers were careful to only drink this water and not the filthy water that they would stand in, sometimes knee-deep, when digging the tunnel.

MINERS' ANEMIA

The workers' symptoms were well known among a handful of professions, giving rise to terms like tunnel disease, brickmakers' anemia, and (using an old word for wasting away to skin and bones) miners' cachexia.

We know now that these are the symptoms of hookworm disease. Once inside a person's intestines, the worms attach to the intestinal wall and suck blood, little by little. A worker with hundreds of the half-inch worms can lose two cups of blood every day, as the worms nourish themselves and grow, the whole time laying eggs to be passed in the feces with the possibility of finding another victim.

Leached of their blood, the workers slowly turned pale or even (to some eyes) greenish. Blood does more than give a pink tinge to your skin; it also supplies your muscles and organs. People who lost blood to hookworm infection thus had anemia: blood loss that left them pale, weak, and far too thin.

But at the time, the dots weren't all connected. Sick people had worms, worms laid eggs. That doesn't mean that the worms were what made the people sick; maybe, some argued, they just took advantage of a weak body. After all, miners spend their time in cramped, filthy conditions, which cause all kinds of disease. They would probably get sick with or without worms.

Fortunately, this was a golden age for parasitology. A quarter-century earlier, doctors had figured out what hookworms and their eggs look like. That research happened in Egypt, where a quarter of the population seemed to be infected with the worms. The same disease was also found in warm, humid environments—including tropical islands. So what was it doing in a tunnel in the Alps?

It turns out that the tunnel conditions explained that part of the puzzle: temperatures could get up to 100° Fahrenheit, and the water running at the miners' feet kept the whole place humid. Any worm or disease that likes tropical conditions would feel totally at home here.

HOOKWORM MYSTERY SOLVED

How could the workers have been infected when their drinking water was so clean? It turns out that the drinking water doesn't matter. And for that bit of information, we can thank an adventurous parasitologist named Arthur Looss. Looss was trying to prove how *Strongyloides* threadworms could mature in the body, so he drank some of their eggs and analyzed his feces. But instead of finding *Strongyloides* eggs, he found those of *Ancylostoma*—hookworm.

Where could they have come from? He remembered that he had accidentally gotten a drop of solution containing hookworm larvae onto his hand in a past experiment. The spot had itched, and he washed his hand, but apparently the hookworms got through. That explained why he had been feeling so exhausted lately. He was working in Egypt, and chalked up his symptoms to the change in climate.

Intrigued, he now squirted hookworm larvae onto his hand, on purpose. After a minute, he scraped the water droplet off his hand and put it under the microscope. Instead of worm larvae, he found the worms' empty skins. They had molted and burrowed into his hand. He had re-created the "miner's itch" that, until now, hadn't been associated with hookworm infection. He then took thymol, recently discovered to be effective against parasites, to rid himself of the infection.

Hookworms, it turns out, don't care what water you drink. They rely on their larvae (from eggs carried in feces) ending up in contact with the next victim's skin. That might mean that one person poops on the ground, and another later walks through it. In mines and tunnels, workers spend their day far away from any proper bathroom. If you gotta go, you gotta go—and feces would pile up in dank corners. The dirty water at the tunnel diggers' feet contained not just garden-variety filth, but also plenty of hookworm larvae that now had access to the workers' skin.

Inside the body, the hookworms do their own brand of tunneling until they find a blood vessel, then ride the bloodstream to the heart and into the lungs. This irritates the lungs, of course, so the person may wheeze and cough. As they cough, the near-invisible worms end up in the throat and mouth, only to be swallowed with the next swig of clean Alpine water. Now they're inside the digestive tract, and once they reach their goal—the small intestine—they dig in their hooks and settle in. They drink their host's blood and release eggs into the intestine to be flushed away in feces.

After the St. Gotthard tunnel was built, surviving infected workers scattered to their homes, and later ended up in tunnel projects and mines in other parts of Europe—and they took hookworm with them. The hookworm epidemic finally got under control when employers started requiring a stool sample before hiring any workers. Only people who didn't have hookworm were allowed to work in the mines. Deworming treatments helped, too, but the most effective change was just to provide "sanitary facilities" for the workers—even something as simple as a bucket would do the job.

CHAPTER 33

RABIES LOSES ITS BITE

RABIES: PARIS

1885

THE BITE OF A RABID DOG WAS A DEATH SENTENCE—UNTIL ONE SCIENTIST THOUGHT TO USE A VACCINE IN AN UNUSUAL WAY.

DEATH TOLL: Unknown—probably just a few human cases

CAUSED BY: The rabies virus

NOTEWORTHY SYMPTOMS: Fever, seizures, convulsions

FATALITY RATE: 100 percent if untreated

THREAT LEVEL TODAY: Rabies still kills 55,000 people each year in places where dogs aren't regularly vaccinated.

NOTABLE FACT: A vaccine is still our only reliable treatment for rabies.

The oldest of the shepherd boys was just fifteen. He and the six others were watching their sheep in a field when a rabid dog attacked them. The younger boys ran while Jean-Baptiste Jupille confronted the dog with his whip. It bit him on the arm, but he was able to pry its jaws open and tie its foaming muzzle shut. He clonked it over the head with one of his wooden shoes, and drowned the dog in a brook. An autopsy later confirmed that the dog was rabid.

In older times—actually, even a few months before the attack— people would have recognized that Jupille had received a death sentence. Rabies was always fatal. First there would be weeks or maybe months of waiting to see if maybe he had dodged the disease, because sometimes a bite isn't deep enough, or the saliva not infectious enough, to transmit it. But if the boy began to feel a tingling in the scar, then headaches and fever were likely to follow. He would seem to fear water, and he would convulse with seizures as his brain swelled and his body tried in vain to fight the infection. There would be no cure.

But now, there was hope, just a tiny bit of hope. Jupille's multiple bites were probably infected with the mysterious substance that Louis Pasteur had been studying. He was calling it a "virus," from a Latin word meaning "poison." Pasteur hadn't been able to see this mysterious thing under a microscope, but he and the other scientists in his lab had managed to come up with an experimental vaccine for it. So far, it had been tried on just a handful of people. Only one case was publicized, a young boy who survived. That was enough for the mayor of Jupille's village, who fired off a letter to Pasteur.

The scientist wrote back right away, counting down the days: Jupille had been bitten on October fourteenth. The return letter would reach the mayor on the eighteenth. The quickest the boy could arrive would probably be the twentieth, at which point the bites would be six days old. The vaccine's previous, famous success had been with a boy treated three days after he was bitten. Success was uncertain, but if the mayor would buy the boy a ticket to Paris, Pasteur would give the experimental treatment free of charge.

FEAR AND LOATHING

France had recently seen a surge in rabies cases. Back in 1878, there were over 500 cases in dogs, triggering officials to round up and slaughter as many strays as they could find. The canine body count was 4,000. In that time, though, only a small number of people were affected. Rabies was never a disease that passed from person to person as a plague. But it was terrifying, on both a medical and metaphorical level. Your sweet pet dog could turn on you, biting the hand that feeds it and delivering certain death. Mad dogs also had a way of going on rampages. The people who flocked to Pasteur's laboratory sometimes came in groups: four boys who had been attacked in New Jersey; nineteen Russians with serious wounds from a wolf that had had to be dispatched with hatchets.

Everybody who showed symptoms of rabies would die from it, but—as the historical accounts show—not everybody who was bitten by a rabid animal ended up getting sick. The rabies virus works agonizingly slowly, making the victims wait weeks or months to find out if they have the fatal illness. During that time, some may have tried to improve their odds by using medical or magical procedures, such as those found in a list of dubious cures that had been compiled by Pliny the Elder, a scholar in ancient Rome. One of those cures specified inserting ashes into the wound, obtained by burning the hair of the dog that bit the patient.

By Pasteur's time, then-modern medicine had ruled out the magical cures. Among the few things that were known to help: cauterization of wounds, with heat or with caustic chemicals. As a boy, Pasteur had watched a group of people drag a mauled man into a blacksmith's shop to have wounds all over his torso seared with a red-hot iron. Even children who had been bitten on the face would have their wounds cauterized. The procedure may have killed some of the virus, but we know today that washing with soap and water works just as well.

CONQUERING THE VIRUS

Pasteur had already built a distinguished career before beginning work on rabies; he had discovered that bacteria were what spoiled milk and wine, and invented a process that was later called pasteurization. He had developed a vaccine for the bacterial disease of chicken cholera. Later, probably recognizing what a headline-grabber it could be, Pasteur turned his attention to rabies.

Thanks to the surge in rabies cases, an army veterinarian had been collecting rabid dogs to study. He happily gave Pasteur two of the frothing animals. Pasteur and his team, including microbiologist Émile Roux, were able to weaken the rabies virus so that it was less deadly—but that also made it useless as a vaccine. Dog bites were so rare, it didn't make sense to vaccinate people before they were bitten. What they needed was a virus that was harmless but that could act quickly, racing against the live rabies.

The team came up with a fast-acting virus, and Roux figured out how to weaken it by taking an infected rabbit's spinal cord and drying it out for weeks. The first test case, a boy named Joseph Meister who had been bitten by a grocer's dog, was subjected to a series of thirteen shots over ten days. He lived, and based on his case, others like Jupille began to show up at Pasteur's door. Today, a version of the same vaccine—in just four doses—is the only reliable treatment for people who have been bitten by a rabid animal.

The treatment worked for Jupille. Pasteur convinced the Institut de France to give him a 1,000 franc prize for his heroism, so he went home both healthy and rich. While Meister had been treated quietly and cautiously, Jupille's story was told more freely, with the press praising his courage. The boy became a minor celebrity.

A statue of Jupille still stands at the Pasteur Institute, immortalized in the moment when the dog clamped on to his arm. Moments like that would soon transition from fateful to mundane, as Pasteur's vaccine became the standard treatment for the bite of a rabid dog. As the vaccine became widespread, rabies lost much of its bite.

CHAPTER 34

THE BERIBERI BOX

BERIBERI: JAPAN
1884

THE JAPANESE NAVY FOUND THAT MANY OF ITS SAILORS WERE WEAK IN THE KNEES—LITERALLY. THE CULPRIT TURNED OUT TO BE NOT AN INFECTION, BUT A PROBLEM WITH THEIR DIET.

DEATH TOLL: About 50 per year in the Japanese navy, but many more sailors were temporarily disabled while on long deployments.

CAUSED BY: Lack of thiamin (vitamin B_1) in the diet

NOTEWORTHY SYMPTOMS: Numb, weak extremities

FATALITY RATE: 100 percent if untreated

THREAT LEVEL TODAY: Beriberi still occurs today in famines and among alcoholics (who have trouble absorbing thiamin).

NOTABLE FACT: Barley-based rations, fed to prisoners to save money, turned out to be healthier than the white rice that soldiers and sailors were given.

Beriberi was a puzzle, but more than that, it was a major logistical problem for the Japanese army and navy. How could you fight when a quarter or a third of your men were weakened or even paralyzed?

The disease had been described in ancient times, and the Japanese knew it well. Their name for it was *kakke*, but they recognized it was the same disease internationally known by the name it had in southeast Asia: beriberi. The name reportedly means, in the Sinhalese language, "I can't, I can't."

Beriberi is a nutritional deficiency. Just as scurvy results from a lack of vitamin C, beriberi comes from a lack of vitamin B_1, better known as thiamin. That wasn't understood at the time, and it was very hard to get the scientific community onboard with the idea of a deficiency.

According to a seventh-century Chinese medical text, the *Essential Formulas for Emergencies Worth a Thousand Pieces of Gold*, beriberi was caused by a poison that emanated from the ground. It would attack the feet first, making them weak and numb, then proceed up the legs and finally reach the chest, causing shortness of breath. If it reaches this stage, the text said, you will die. Whatever the cause, nobody had a good answer for how to cure it: not the Japanese with acupuncture needles, and not the British, with their penchant for bloodletting. In the 1880s, the best bet would be to look for an infectious disease—some kind of germ.

THE EXPERIMENT

The new navy surgeon Kanehiro Takaki wasn't buying the poison theory. He remembered a story his father, an Imperial Palace Guard, had told him. Beriberi was rampant among the guards, and they believed it had something to do with the food they were issued. The provisions box, Takaki later recalled, was nicknamed the "beriberi box."

Around 1850, Japan began to trade more with the Western world. Deciding it needed a military, Japan had British shipyards build British-style ships for the country's new navy, which it mirrored after Britain's. The newly founded army also looked to the West, but used the German military as its model. Perhaps because of this split, the navy solved the beriberi problem much sooner than the army did.

Takaki was determined to find out why so much of the navy was succumbing to beriberi, a disease that the British never suffered from. They sailed in the same seas, in similar if not identical boats. If the cause came from the environment, it should affect both nationalities equally. The swampy soil idea was a nonstarter since the disease often struck sailors who hadn't been on land in months. People with and without beriberi could share quarters without transmitting the disease, so he crossed infection off his list. Incidence of the disease varied by rank, but what could that signify?

Nutrition science was in its infancy. Vitamins and minerals were unknown, although some Europeans had stumbled on cures for scurvy without entirely understanding why they worked. Scientists of the time had recently figured out that food was made of carbohydrate, fat, and protein, and they knew that a lack of protein can make people weak.

Takaki suspected that the navy's problem was in its rations. One of the few differences between the higher- and lower-ranked sailors, among the warships whose records Takaki examined, was their food. Sailors were given plain rice to eat, plus supplemental "ration money," and could purchase other items for a fee. Officers had no problem filling out their diets, but lower-ranked sailors, saving money to send home, sometimes attempted to subsist entirely on the free rice.

The results were disastrous. In 1883, a group of 276 cadets left on a nine-month training voyage that traveled to New Zealand and Hawaii. During the trip, 169 of them came down with beriberi, and 25 died. Takaki secured funding to send the 1884 voyage out with enhanced rations, including meat and condensed milk. He thought that the increased protein would stave off beriberi.

He was wrong about the protein, but right about the result of the richer diet. On this voyage, nobody died, and there were only 14 cases of the disease. The sick men were the ones who had refused to eat parts of the enhanced rations, such as the meat and milk.

The navy switched all of its men to the more nutritious diet, and beriberi became rare again. By 1887, there were only three cases of beriberi in the entire navy.

PICKY CHICKENS

The army, meanwhile, refused to believe that changing soldiers' diets would do anything to help the 25 percent of soldiers who suffered from nerve damage or worse. But the army couldn't help noticing that some civilian prisons had eliminated beriberi by the cost-saving measure of mixing prisoners' rice with cheaper grains like barley. In 1885 barley was included in soldiers' rations, and beriberi rates fell.

The strongest evidence for beriberi as a thiamin deficiency came from someone who was trying very, very hard to prove that it was an infectious disease. Christiaan Eijkman was a Dutch scientist doing his experiments on a military base in Indonesia. He acquired a flock of chickens, and began injecting half of them with the blood of beriberi victims. For the longest time, none of them came down with the disease.

Then all of a sudden, birds started developing weakness in their legs. The problem was that it was affecting chickens in both groups. Suspecting that one chicken had infected another, he bought new, uninfected chickens and kept them in separate cages. They still developed the disease. He started a new lab in another location, but chickens kept there also developed the disease. Eijkman prepared to do even more experiments on the chickens but then, all of a sudden, all of the chickens recovered.

It turned out to be the food. For five months, the person who fed the chickens had been getting day-old rice from the cook at the base. The mess hall then got a new head cook, who refused to give away the leftover rice. So the lab switched back to the usual feed, a brown rice bought at the market.

Eijkman conducted one experiment after another to figure out what was so different between the cooked white rice, which caused beriberi, and the raw brown rice, which did not. Slowly the answer emerged: to stay healthy, the chickens needed to eat the brown part of the rice, the part that is "polished" off to produce white rice. The rice polishings could be added back to the diet, though, curing the illness at will. It took years to convince the scientific community—and even for Eijkman to convince himself—that there really was something special about the polishings. But the discovery turned out to be spot-on: the rice polishings were full of what we now know as B vitamins.

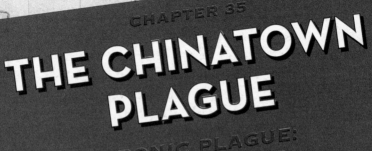

CHAPTER 35

THE CHINATOWN PLAGUE

BUBONIC PLAGUE: SAN FRANCISCO

1900

A CASE OF PLAGUE IN SAN FRANCISCO'S CHINATOWN TRIGGERED A BIZARRE, ILLOGICAL QUARANTINE.

DEATH TOLL: 191 in San Francisco between 1900 and 1908

CAUSED BY: The bacterium *Yersinia pestis*

NOTEWORTHY SYMPTOMS: Swollen lymph nodes ("buboes") in groin, armpits, or neck

FATALITY RATE: 60 percent is typical for bubonic plague

THREAT LEVEL TODAY: Low. Plague is rare, and can be treated with antibiotics if caught in time. A handful of cases still occur in America each year.

NOTABLE FACT: The plague didn't last long in humans, but made the leap to squirrels and other wild rodents, where it still persists today.

When Wing Chung Ging died in a San Francisco boarding-house in 1900, he was the first official plague case ever in the mainland United States.

Outbreaks of plague had been raging in Asia for decades: Hong Kong, Canton, and India were hard hit. Just as in centuries before, the plague bacteria seemed to travel by ship rat. The disease spread across Asia and then the world, one high-traffic seaport at a time.

We don't know how Wing Chung Ging contracted plague. He didn't bring it from China; he had lived in San Francisco for six-teen years before he died. Perhaps the source was a ship that came from Hong Kong in 1899, with two cases of plague onboard. The ship was quarantined at nearby Angel Island. A search turned up eleven stowaways, but two escaped, and were found later in the bay—dead of plague.

Wing Chung Ging died in the boardinghouse shortly after mid-night. A man sleeping in a nearby bed notified the night clerk, who turned the body over to city officials. A pathologist examined the body in the wee hours of the morning, and when he realized this was no ordinary death, he called in two higher-ups. That after-noon, the city's senior health officer announced that a possible case of plague had been found, and the Chinese portion of the city was under quarantine until scientists could confirm whether it truly was plague or not.

A bacteriologist would take the dead man's lymph glands to the laboratory at Angel Island, and attempt to grow bacteria from them in broth. The results would be injected into experimental animals to see if they developed the symptoms of plague. But the process would take several days, with Chinese citizens essentially under house arrest and the whole city wondering if the Black Death had come to town. The *San Francisco Chronicle* wrote that "[a] chat-tering monkey in the death cell of the federal laboratory on Angel Island holds the fate of San Francisco within its mangy little hide."

THE PLAGUE GERM DISCOVERED

Officials in San Francisco were working with half an understanding of plague. They didn't know that rats and fleas were involved in its spread, but the bacteria that cause plague had been freshly discovered. Just six years earlier, in 1894, two scientists had extracted the tiny killer from the buboes of plague victims in Hong Kong.

The first scientist was the revered Shibasaburo Kitasato, who arrived in Hong Kong with a team of experts. The superintendent of the Civil Hospital there gave him prime laboratory space and allowed him to take samples from dead patients' bodies without their families' consent. Kitasato worked quickly, announcing his findings after just a few days' work. His published description partially matches what we know today about *Yersinia pestis*. Some of the details, though, aren't quite right.

The second scientist was Alexandre Yersin, who arrived later, and got a less friendly reception. He didn't have Kitasato's funding or diplomatic connections, and initially was not given access to patients. Yersin built his own laboratory in a grass hut next to the hospital, and obtained his first samples by bribing a cemetery guard to look the other way while he sliced buboes off corpses about to be buried.

Yersin suggested the name *Pasteurella pestis*, after the Pasteur Institute where he had studied. Decades later it was renamed *Yersinia pestis* in his honor. Although Yersin didn't receive much credit for his discovery at the time, later work showed that his report was accurate, while Kitasato had probably described a mixture that included the plague bacterium and another germ.

UNFAIR QUARANTINE

In 1900, the San Francisco health department was working with this new knowledge. Gone were the debates about whether plague was transmitted by a "miasma" or by the breath or sight of a victim. Disease after disease was unveiled to be caused by a germ—tuberculosis, cholera, and now plague. If the bacterium entered your body, you could get sick.

But nobody in the city understood how the germ got from person to person. Many of the people of San Francisco thought that plague was a natural consequence of filth. Chinatown, like other slum areas of the city, certainly had filth in abundance.

The quarantine around Chinatown was likely directed as much by xenophobia as by mere ignorance. Chinese immigrants faced massive discrimination, starting with their ability to enter the country at all. When plague was found in Chinatown, the newspapers exploded with blame. During the quarantine, Chinese residents were banned from leaving the area to go to work in other parts of the city or even to buy food. White residents, however, were allowed to cross the quarantine line freely, thus making it not really a quarantine.

Wing Chung Ging's death was confirmed as plague, but only a handful of other cases ever appeared. The plague fizzled out.

THE PLAGUE REVISITS

In 1906 a second wave of plague hit San Francisco. By then, however, city officials were thinking more clearly. Maybe the improvement was due to the racial makeup of the victims—this one occurred outside the Chinese area and struck mostly white Americans. But the other important difference is that rats had been found guilty of spreading plague.

The clues had been there all along. Europeans had noted that dead rats could be found in cities afflicted with plague. Sometimes the hypothesis was that the rats had caught plague from the humans; other times that people caught plague from whiffs of the miasma created by piles of dead rats. With a germ to blame, though, there were fewer dots to connect. People now had to find how the bacterium traveled from person to person. It might be airborne, like measles, or fecal-oral, like cholera. Both Yersin and

Kitasato found plague bacteria in the dirt floors of plague victims' houses in Hong Kong. Could that be the cause?

One of Yersin's colleagues, Paul-Louis Simond, investigated the suspicion that fleas and rats might be involved. In a famous experiment, he placed a healthy rat in a wire cage suspended next to a rat that was dying of plague. Fleas jumped from the dead rat to the live one, and soon the living rat, too, was a dead rat. Others expanded on this work, and soon the rat's role in plague transmission was an acknowledged fact.

And so when the plague came to San Francisco the second time, the story centered not on the presumed filth of immigrants, but on the new villain of plague: the rat. People put tight lids on their garbage cans, and children were paid a bounty for every dead rat they could turn in. The outbreak did not last long.

CHAPTER 36

DOWN BY THE RIVERSIDE

SLEEPING SICKNESS: UGANDA

1901

THIS PARASITE FROM A FLY BITE BURROWS INTO YOUR BRAIN AND CAN ALTER THE BRAIN'S FUNCTIONS. SLEEPING AT THE WRONG TIME OF DAY IS A MILD SYMPTOM COMPARED TO THE CONFUSION AND VIOLENT IMPULSES THAT PLAGUE VICTIMS IN THE MORE ADVANCED STAGES.

DEATH TOLL: 250,000 in the Busoga region of Uganda

CAUSED BY: Protozoan parasites in the genus *Trypanosoma*

NOTEWORTHY SYMPTOMS: Disturbed brain function and sleep cycles

FATALITY RATE: 100 percent if untreated

THREAT LEVEL TODAY: This disease is still around, and affects 30,000 people per year.

NOTABLE FACT: Domestic animals, like most breeds of horses and cattle, can also be affected by sleeping sickness.

Around 1900, after the British poked their colonial noses into Uganda and changed many aspects of the economy and the environment, an epidemic of sleeping sickness broke out in the Busoga region, at the northern tip of Lake Victoria.

Sleeping sickness sounds cozy; however, it's anything but. In the first stage of the disease, the person has some mild, boring symptoms: fever, achy joints, itchiness. Since the disease is transmitted by the bite of the tsetse fly, not much bigger than a housefly, a person in the first stage may also have a fly bite that turns into a raw wound. But soon enough, that goes away.

The second stage is the scary one. After a while (how long depends on which strain of sleeping sickness ended up infecting you), the disease reaches the brain. The protozoan parasite, or trypanosome, burrows into the brain and starts disturbing precious functions. A person in this stage of the disease may become confused or violent. One sufferer, speaking on a video for Doctors Without Borders (a group that treats the disease today in remote African villages), said that he thought he was under some kind of evil spell because all of a sudden he couldn't recognize his own wife and son.

It's in this second stage, as the person approaches death, that the disease earns its name. The parasite doesn't make you more sleepy, but it does interfere with the part of the brain that keeps track of what time of day it is. A person with sleeping sickness takes restless naps throughout the day and night.

Africans living in the tsetse-fly belt, which makes up more than a third of the continent, have customs that would seem to reduce their chance of getting sleeping sickness. For example, a village in the middle of a forest traditionally has a large cleared area around it that is consistently kept up. This keeps enemies and forest animals from preying at the back door. It also has the side effect of eliminating tsetse fly habitat.

However, when the British came in to establish a colony, they forced people to move to new areas and levied taxes that required the people to carve out more land from the forest for agriculture.

The forest, it seems, fought back. British and Africans alike became victims of a new surge in cases of sleeping sickness.

Corkscrew-shaped parasites had been found in fish, frogs, and mice, but they were just curiosities until they were connected with a wasting disease of horses and cattle in India called *surra*. A smear of the sick animals' blood, put under a microscope, also showed the corkscrew-like parasite. Back in Africa, Scottish bacteriologist David Bruce was trying to track down the disease that killed all of the horses and cows that British colonists would fruitlessly bring to Africa. The Zulu called the disease *nagana*, meaning something like "laziness." It, too, was caused by a corkscrew-shaped parasite. These related species were later named trypanosomes.

BITE OF THE FLY

We now know that sleeping sickness is essentially the human version of nagana, and it's spread by a tsetse fly. These flies live in forests, resting on tree trunks and feeding on whatever large animal wanders by. Females don't bother laying eggs; they grow a single larva inside their body, and when it is ready to turn into an adult, the mother gives birth to it on the forest floor, ideally on moist soil under some low-lying plants, perhaps on the bank of a pond. The larva immediately burrows and forms its pupa, and soon afterward is able to emerge as an adult fly.

This strategy puts tsetse flies on the banks of ponds and rivers, and anywhere forest meets open areas in the right climate. If a village is built in a humid area without a buffer of empty land to keep the forest at bay, that village's border is an ideal place for tsetse flies. Same goes for the clearings in forests that are used as cemeteries or as sacred shrines. What's more, a lot of the cash crops Africans began farming to pay colonial taxes also made prime tsetse territory. Those include banana, mango, sugar, and cocoa plantations, not to mention Uganda's biggest export today, coffee.

The British sent researchers to figure out the nagana epidemic, and later, sleeping sickness. Researchers paid "fly boys" to walk through assigned areas, counting how many flies landed on them. They published reports giving statistics such as how many flies could be found in a given area "per fly-boy per mile." They began destroying areas of forest to remove the flies' habitat.

And just a few years into the effort, in 1904, the first medication was discovered that was able to help people with sleeping sickness: atoxyl, an arsenic compound. Basically, the trypanosomes that had made it to the brain could be poisoned with arsenic. That made atoxyl a dangerous drug, and sometimes people died from arsenic poisoning. But it was worth a try for someone afflicted with the second stage of sleeping sickness. Without the new drugs, the disease was always fatal.

Today, less-toxic drugs are available, and humanitarian organizations like Doctors Without Borders are attempting to stamp out the disease for good. They offer screening tests to figure out who might be carrying the parasite without knowing it, and treat them to kill the parasite. That means one more person that the flies can't pick up the parasite from—an important step in removing the disease from the area.

CHAPTER 37

TYPHOID MARY AND FRIENDS

TYPHOID FEVER: NEW YORK

1907

MARY FELT PERFECTLY HEALTHY, BUT STILL MANAGED TO INFECT OTHER PEOPLE WITH TYPHOID FEVER. SHE WAS ONE OF MANY HEALTHY CARRIERS OF THE DISEASE, BUT THE ONLY ONE IMPRISONED AS A RESULT.

DEATH TOLL: 1 from Typhoid Mary (lifetime total); 12,670 from typhoid in the United States in 1907

CAUSED BY: The bacterium *Salmonella enterica* subsp. *enterica* serovar Typhi

NOTEWORTHY SYMPTOMS: Abdominal pain, weakness, constipation

FATALITY RATE: 10 percent or more

THREAT LEVEL TODAY: High in places without good sanitation; low elsewhere

NOTABLE FACT: Cooking kills typhoid, but Mary's signature dish was an uncooked one: ice cream with fresh peaches.

There were thousands of Typhoid Marys in the United States in 1907, but only one ended up imprisoned for life. She was responsible for one death and more than two dozen illnesses, even though she herself was never sick. This is the story of typhoid fever's healthy carriers.

Mary Mallon's part begins in the summer of 1906, when she cooked for a wealthy New York family vacationing in Oyster Bay, Long Island. Six people in the household got sick in the space of a week, while living in a rented house. The owner of the house, afraid he would never be able to rent it again, called in a sanitation engineer named George Soper. He would investigate.

Typhoid fever is no relation to typhus. Typhus is a louse-borne disease more often associated with starving soldiers than posh vacationers. For example, typhus caused many of the fatalities in Napoleon's ill-fated invasion of Russia. Typhoid fever, on the other hand, is a form of salmonella transmitted by feces. Typhoid got its name because it shares symptoms with typhus. Both cause abdominal pain and a fever that can last for weeks.

To come down with typhoid fever, you need to ingest some of the bacteria, which then break into your intestinal cells and hitch a ride around your body, multiplying in white blood cells before making a home in the gallbladder. Whenever the gallbladder squirts bile into the intestines, typhoid bacteria are squirted too.

Common ways to get typhoid are through contaminated water, or from a typhoid patient's unwashed hands. The health department had already ruled out the family's food and milk. The water supply tested clean, even when fluorescent dye was added to the stables and cesspools in the area; clearly nothing was leaking into the well. Soper tracked down the source of the family's favorite food, soft clams, and found that they had been harvested from places that were polluted with sewage. But that theory collapsed when he realized the dates didn't match up: the family ate clams in July but didn't get sick until the end of August.

Did anything unusual happen in early August, he asked? It turns out that was when the family brought in a new cook, Mary Mallon. She left shortly after the outbreak. Soper managed to track down Mallon's employment history. She had been with a family that got sick in 1900, where the laundress was the first to suffer. The family blamed the outbreak on the laundress. She had gone with a lawyer's family to a cottage in Maine, where another outbreak happened. Her resume read like a catalog of epidemics, always in affluent families. Typhoid had followed Mallon to seven of the eight households Soper found she had worked in.

Then the trail went cold—Mallon hadn't been seen since the Long Island outbreak—so Soper just kept an ear out for reports of typhoid among the rich. Soon enough, he found Mallon in a house with a fresh typhoid outbreak. The family's daughter died, and now Mallon was associated with a body count.

ISOLATION

Mary Mallon was at work, feeling perfectly healthy, when George Soper came to tell her she was giving people typhoid, and needed to provide samples of her urine and feces. She told him the truth: that she had never been sick with typhoid, and that he had no right to harass her at work. So Soper turned the case over to the Department of Health, which sent Dr. Sara Josephine Baker. Maybe Mallon would respond better to a woman's request. And Dr. Baker took five police officers with her, in case she didn't.

As Dr. Baker tells it, Mallon threatened her with a carving fork, then disappeared in the commotion. The police followed her footprints through the snow to another house, where they spotted a flash of blue cloth under the stairs that led up to the front door, behind a pile of ash cans. "She came out fighting and swearing," Dr. Baker wrote later. "She knew she had never had typhoid fever. She was maniacal in her integrity." Dr. Baker wrestled her into the ambulance, and sat on her for the ride to the hospital.

For the next three years, authorities held Mallon at a hospital on North Brother Island within sight of Manhattan. They took blood, urine, and stool samples; 120 of 163 tested positive for typhoid. Mallon still didn't believe she was sick, and sent her own samples to an independent lab. Results came back negative. She threatened and pleaded, and eventually she brought a lawsuit, which she lost. In 1910, New York City got a new health commissioner, Ernst Lederle. He ordered her release. "For heaven's sake," he said to a reporter for the *New York American*, "can't the poor creature be given a chance to live?"

HEALTHY CARRIERS

Healthy carriers of typhoid were not a new discovery, although Mallon was the first one New York City's health department had been asked to deal with. Just twelve years earlier, the army had undertaken a massive study of typhoid and how to prevent its spread.

The study came thanks to the Spanish-American War, where battlefield death counts were dwarfed by the number of soldiers who died in training camps back home. A thorough investigation found that soldiers were getting sick from fecal germs that spread through the camp in many ways: flies landing in open latrines and then on food, for example, or orderlies at field hospitals who would take care of typhoid patients and then return to their bunks with unwashed hands.

The army investigators found that a soldier who contracted typhoid could shed the germs in his feces for weeks before showing symptoms, and for weeks after he recovered. Some seemed to be contagious for life. And some were contagious even though they never came down with typhoid fever at all.

There were hundreds if not thousands of healthy carriers already on the streets of New York City, the number likely growing by 100 per year. Doctors and public health officials debated what to do with these people. It wouldn't be possible to round them all up; it wouldn't be ethical to keep them away from their families and livelihood; and it would all be too expensive anyway. New York's health board wrote a guideline that said carriers just had to keep their address on file, and had to promise not to work in a food-handling job. Mary Mallon signed her affidavit, and went to work in a laundry.

Five years later, authorities investigated an outbreak at a maternity hospital and found a familiar face working there as cook. Mallon was shipped off to North Brother Island again, this time for good. Meanwhile, other healthy carriers broke their promises and were allowed to stay at home. Acquitting a restaurant owner, one judge wrote: "I could not legally sentence this man to jail on account of his health."

Mallon may have been under special scrutiny because her case was already famous; the newspapers had christened her "Typhoid Mary." The health officers may have held a personal grudge about Mallon's combative attitude, or they may have been biased against Irish immigrants, a common sentiment of the time. Mallon was also at a disadvantage as a single woman. Men who carried typhoid often received a stipend to support their families while they trained for new jobs. Whatever the reason, Mary Mallon would never leave the island. She died on North Brother Island at the age of sixty-nine. She had spent twenty-six years in exile.

CHAPTER 38

AN UNPOPULAR DISCOVERY

PELLAGRA: MISSISSIPPI
1914

SOUTHERN POLITICIANS WERE EAGER TO SOLVE THE PROBLEM OF PELLAGRA— UNTIL THE CAUSE TURNED OUT TO BE POVERTY.

DEATH TOLL: Estimated at 100,000 over 40 years

CAUSED BY: Lack of niacin (vitamin B_3) in the diet

NOTEWORTHY SYMPTOMS: Rough, blistering skin on the neck and hands, diarrhea, dementia

FATALITY RATE: 64 percent in some institutions

THREAT LEVEL TODAY: Low except in famine situations.

NOTABLE FACT: The disease especially struck two groups of people: Americans eating little more than grits and cornbread, and Italians relying on corn-based polenta.

A poor Georgia man with hookworm was the first clue that the American South might have a pellagra problem. As his doctor reported in a 1902 issue of the *Journal of Tropical Medicine*, the man had all the symptoms of pellagra, a disease so far only known to affect poor farmers in Italy who had nothing better to eat than cornmeal polenta.

This man was only twenty-nine, and for half of his life he had the same symptoms every spring. He would become thirsty, weak, and depressed, and his hands and the tops of his feet would break out in blisters. By July he would feel better, and then the cycle would repeat the next year. He had hookworms, sure, but he'd been having his problems for longer than hookworms are known to live. With medication he passed 600 worms, but the pellagra symptoms continued.

"If he [has] pellagra, the disease is so far advanced that nothing can be done for him," the doctor wrote. "He has been advised to go to a cooler climate, and to be careful not to eat decomposed Indian corn." This was the best advice the doctor had, based on what was known of the disease from Italy. There, under names like *mal de rosa* (after the color of the irritated skin) or Alpine scurvy, it affected the poorest of the poor in corn-growing regions. Traditionally these people ate porridge made from barley, farro, or spelt, but corn and potatoes from the Americas turned out to be cheaper. Early reports likened the disease to leprosy, because the blisters on the hands and chest give way to thickened skin. It clustered in poor families, but the Italian doctors quickly concluded that it was not contagious and not inherited. Its cause was the corn.

Today, we know that pellagra develops when people don't have enough niacin (vitamin B_3) in their diet. Processed cornmeal is missing that vitamin. The Italian scientists debated whether corn was missing something that's essential for people to have, or whether it contained a toxin that caused the disease. But American doctors and scientists ended up having an entirely different debate.

ON THE CASE

The epidemic soon exploded. Reports began to come from mental hospitals, orphanages, and other institutions. Some had no pellagra, but others had dozens or hundreds of cases. Between 1907 and 1911, eight southern states reported over 15,000 cases of pellagra, with a fatality rate of nearly 40 percent.

Doctors learned to look for the "three Ds": dermatitis, diarrhea, and dementia. The characteristic skin rash was sensitive to light, so it would blister and roughen skin surfaces that were exposed to light—mainly the hands, and a "necklace" pattern around the shirt collar. The symptoms appeared in the spring, after a lean winter spent eating little but grits and cornbread.

A national conference on pellagra in South Carolina featured speeches from the governor, a senator, and the superintendent of the State Hospital for the Insane, where many cases had been reported. Seventy-two physicians were in attendance. The next year, they held the conference again, and the crowd of doctors had ballooned to 394.

At first, government officials in the affected states were eager to solve the problem. This was the age of discovery for infectious diseases: plague, malaria, and typhus were all understood as the work of specific, contagious organisms. Several southern states formed pellagra commissions. Mississippi, Tennessee, and North Carolina requested federal aid. Philanthropists gave donations. Atlanta opened the first hospital dedicated to pellagra. Pretty soon, it seemed, the problem would be licked. The U.S. surgeon general appointed an epidemiologist named Joseph Goldberger to figure out what was going on. He didn't find evidence of an infectious disease, but rather a dietary one. In the institutions with high rates of pellagra, only patients or inmates had the disease, not staff. He figured that more nutritious food, including milk and beans, could prevent pellagra but would cost $700 a year for each institution. He secured funding to try the improved diet in two orphanages that had 172 cases of pellagra between them. When spring came around, only one child relapsed, and there were no new cases. When the funding ran out, pellagra returned with a vengeance.

To drive the point home, Goldberger convinced the governor to pardon a group of convicts at the pellagra-free Rankin Farm at the Mississippi State Penitentiary in exchange for volunteering for his experiment. Goldberger kept the subjects in a building with mosquito-proof screens, and fed them a monotonous, corn-based diet all summer. After six months, half of them had pellagra. "I have been through a thousand hells," one of the convicts said. Critics accused Goldberger of torture, and said they still didn't believe the disease was anything other than infectious. Goldberger, exasperated, conducted his most disgusting, but convincing, trial.

In a series of experiments, a group of doctors including Goldberger injected themselves with blood collected from pellagra patients on their deathbeds. They mixed flakes from skin lesions into dough balls along with samples of urine and diarrhea from the patients. After somehow choking these down, they experienced nothing more serious than stomach upset.

"THE NATION MUST SAVE ITS OWN"

The southern doctors and politicians who were so eager to solve the pellagra epidemic changed their tune when it looked like the disease was not contagious, but dietary. More than that, it occurred in people who were underfed, either deliberately or because they lived in poor families that couldn't afford anything better than the "three M" diet of meat (fatback pork), meal (that is, corn grits), and molasses. In other words, the epidemic of pellagra was an epidemic of poverty.

President Warren Harding promised to take action, writing to the surgeon general that, "Famine and plague are words almost foreign to our American vocabulary . . . The nation could not wait a single day to take action. It must save its own." But the southern states were no longer onboard. Representative James Byrnes wrote to the president refusing the promised Red Cross aid, and demanding an apology for accusing his state of harboring famine and plague.

The problem wasn't truly solved until years later, when a group of hunting dogs (kept hungry to make them better hunters) developed the canine form of the disease, called black tongue. A supplement of yeast cured them, and later, the pellagra-preventing factor—known briefly as vitamin PP—was found to be niacin.

Why had the pellagra epidemic come so quickly, then, if corn was a staple for centuries? The reason seemed to be a new processing technique that separated the parts of the corn kernel, discarding the parts that contained niacin. Traditional cooking techniques, on the other hand—including the process that makes corn tortillas and posole—involved using the whole corn grain and softening it in alkaline water, which has the side effect of making the niacin more available for digestion.

The pellagra problem went away in the 1940s. A 1941 law required bread and flour to be fortified with thiamin, niacin, and iron. World War II rationing brought awareness of eating a quality diet, and war-effort jobs lifted people out of poverty a little.

CHAPTER 39

THE "SPANISH" FLU

INFLUENZA: WORLDWIDE

1918

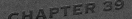

THIS OUTBREAK OF FLU TURNED DEADLY, KILLING MORE PEOPLE THAN THE WAR ITSELF DID. IT STRUCK THE YOUNG AND HEALTHY, LEAVING THEIR DECEASED BODIES A DISCOLORED SHADE OF BLUE.

DEATH TOLL: At least 50 million people, or about 3 percent of the world's population

CAUSED BY: The influenza A virus, subtype H1N1

NOTEWORTHY SYMPTOMS: Fever, pneumonia, and skin that appears blue at death

FATALITY RATE: 2.5 percent (compared to 0.1 percent in ordinary flu)

THREAT LEVEL TODAY: High. International authorities keep a close watch on influenza outbreaks to spot the next potential pandemic before it happens.

NOTABLE FACT: Unlike typical strains of influenza, this flu mostly struck down the young and healthy.

Influenza struck everywhere in 1918, but at first only Spain was free to talk about it. As a neutral party in World War I, its newspapers weren't concerned with whether reporting on illness would make the country appear weak. German and Austrian governments didn't want to let on that their soldiers were being struck down with an unusually brutal flu; neither did French and English forces. One of the earliest outbreaks, in Kansas early that year, was published in a government public health report but not the local newspaper.

The flu would begin with the usual fevers, headache, and weakness. But rather than recovering, some of its victims would end up with discolored skin, which the doctors described as "heliotrope cyanosis" after a pretty purple flower. Lung infection often followed, so that the early death certificates often just listed pneumonia.

By the time the war ended and soldiers began returning home, Spain was settled in many minds as the source of the epidemic: it was the "Spanish flu" or the "Spanish lady." In Spain, the disease was nicknamed the Naples Soldier, after a musical number that an actor quipped was as catchy as the flu. That song came from an operetta based on the Don Juan story, which became a metaphor for the disease. (A cartoon in the Spanish newspaper *El Imparcial* shows a microbe in a cape, quoting Don Juan: "I scaled palace walls, I descended upon cottages . . .")

By the end of 1918, long before the era of easy air travel, the microbe had scaled walls and crossed borders all over the world. The Associated Press reported that in India, "hospitals are so choked, it is impossible to remove the dead to make room for the dying." Native Alaskans' villages were sometimes wiped out completely. The flu struck so many places so quickly that tracking its spread was impossible. Even today, epidemiologists argue. Perhaps it began in that Kansas military base, where cases began as early as January or February in a nearby town.

Or maybe the flu really began in China, where the death toll wasn't nearly as severe. The Chinese may have had protection from an earlier variant of the same disease, and the virus could have mutated as it migrated. England and France imported Chinese laborers to free up men for fighting, and the disease could have come with them. Another theory holds that an Allied military camp at Étaples was the source, with outbreaks of a harsh flu as early as 1916. The Chinese laborers then could have taken the disease home with them, rather than the other way around.

NOT "JUST" THE FLU

This was more than an ordinary flu. In an average year, the flu is still capable of killing. It typically carries off more than a few children, elderly people, and those who had other health problems to start with. Even healthy people who brush off the initial symptoms as "just the flu" often quickly find that it's not a trifling infection.

The pattern of deaths in 1918 brought another mystery: the flu was killing healthy young adults at a much higher rate than anyone else. The elderly may have had a secret weapon: anyone over seventy years old may have had some protection from a previous pandemic. But that still doesn't explain why a twenty-year-old man would have slimmer chances at surviving than, say, a child. One explanation came later: what was called the "cytokine storm." Cytokines are chemical signals that our bodies use to summon immune cells to the places they're needed. In some deadly infections, the body produces so many cytokines that the immune system ends up destroying healthy tissue. In these rare cases, a healthy immune system can backfire on its owner.

But why would this flu be different from other years? Recently, scientists were able to reconstruct the virus's DNA thanks to bodies that had been buried in permafrost and never fully decayed. The deadly flu, it turns out, was descended from an avian, or bird, flu. Influenza viruses can live in a bird's digestive system without causing any significant symptoms. But with a few tweaks to its genetic code, a flu virus can learn how to break into a mammal's lung cells. It's also possible for two viruses to combine—for example, in the body of a pig. Whether that happened in 1918, we can't be sure. But this virus was clearly something new to most people's immune systems, and that may be why it was so much more dangerous than other forms of the flu that had come before.

By the end of 1918, the flu had run its course. Three waves came and went, starting with a milder one that conferred immunity on people lucky enough to catch it early. The later waves were more dangerous. But then, the flu began to disappear.

The flu virus mutates quickly, and after causing severe disease it may have mutated on its own to be less virulent. Or perhaps death tolls declined because health care workers got better at recognizing and managing the symptoms and the bacterial infections that would result.

In 2009, a ghost of the 1918 flu arrived. Its "H" and "N" proteins were a match for the 1918 strain: like it, this one was categorized as type A, subtype H1N1. Again, the new virus was more severe than the usual seasonal flu, killing young adults with what looked like a cytokine storm. Public health officials braced for a pandemic. We now have vaccines for influenza, updated each year to reflect the virus's most recent mutations. But in 2009 H1N1 came as a surprise, and wasn't included in the flu shot. Governments rushed to create a vaccine for the new strain, and alerted health workers to be on the lookout for a tough new flu. In the end, the would-be pandemic fizzled. Was it defeated by well-informed public health measures? Or did we just luck out? It's hard to tell.

CHAPTER 40
SERUM BY DOGSLED

DIPHTHERIA: ALASKA
1925

WHEN DIPHTHERIA BROKE OUT IN A REMOTE ALASKA TOWN, THERE SEEMED TO BE NO HOPE OF SAVING THE TOWN'S CHILDREN, UNTIL DOGSLED MUSHERS CAME TO THE RESCUE.

DEATH TOLL: At least 5

CAUSED BY: The bacterium *Corynebacterium diphtheriae*

NOTEWORTHY SYMPTOMS: Sore throat, loss of appetite, fever

FATALITY RATE: 20 percent in children under age five; 10 percent in older children

THREAT LEVEL TODAY: Low. There is an effective vaccine.

NOTABLE FACT: The Iditarod dogsled race follows part of the same trail as the 1925 serum relay.

I t was January when the lone doctor in Nome, Alaska, noticed the gray, leathery coating on a three-year-old's throat. More than a month earlier, a child had died of what seemed like tonsillitis. The doctor had ruled out diphtheria since it tends to occur in sweeping outbreaks, not isolated cases. The following weeks brought a surge in tonsillitis cases, and then another death. Tonsillitis was not usually a fatal disease.

This was in the days before antibiotics, but there was actually a cure for diphtheria: an antitoxin made from the blood of horses. Nome's doctor, Curtis Welch, had a small supply of it, but it had expired the previous summer. He had ordered a replacement shipment, but Nome's port freezes over every winter, and the city became icebound before the serum could arrive.

Dr. Welch feared that giving expired serum to the weak toddler would do more harm than good. The next day, the child died, and a seven-year-old girl turned up with the disease. Dr. Welch gave her a dose of antitoxin, using up almost all of his 8,000-unit supply, but she died anyway.

The port was closed to boats. The airplanes of 1925 could not safely fly in the cold weather. The nearest railroad station was over 600 miles away, a twenty-five-day journey by dogsled. Diphtheria was extremely contagious, and an outbreak could devastate the town by the time any serum could arrive that way.

But it was the only way. Two days after the first diagnosis, Dr. Welch sent telegrams to other Alaska cities warning them not to let anyone travel to Nome. He also sent one to the U.S. Public Health Service in Washington, D.C.: "An epidemic of diphtheria is almost inevitable here STOP I am in urgent need of [many doses] of diphtheria antitoxin STOP Mail is only form of transportation . . ." The mail came by train to the town of Nenana, and then had to cover 674 miles by dogsled. Deliveries normally took thirty days, but the record was nine. Dr. Welch figured the serum could only last six days in the brutal cold.

THE PLAGUE OF CHILDREN

Diphtheria had a way of sweeping into an area and carrying off children, with a 20 percent fatality rate among children under age five. An earlier New England outbreak had been called "the plague of children."

A diphtheria infection can begin when a person breathes in a droplet containing the bacteria, often from an infected person's cough or sneeze. People can be contagious for weeks before developing symptoms. Some people with the bacteria never have symptoms at all, spreading the bacteria unknowingly.

Once in the throat, the bacteria begin creating the leathery membrane Dr. Welch noticed. They make a two-part toxin. One part latches onto a cell in the throat, splitting it open. The other enters the cell, finds the factory that produces proteins the cell needs to survive, and jams that machine. The cells die. Their membranes, their leftover proteins, and rescuing cells from the immune system become glued together with the multiplying bacteria in a thick gray layer. The disease's name comes from the Greek word *diphthera*, "leather." The leathery membrane often forms on the tonsils or in the throat, but it can also grow deep in the lungs or in other parts of the body. If a piece breaks off, it can block the airway, suffocating the child.

In 1925, there was no way to kill the bacteria. The discovery of antibiotics was still years away. But the serum that existed could stop the toxin from doing damage. It was made by growing the diphtheria bacteria in broth, filtering out the bacteria, and injecting small amounts of the toxin-laced liquid into horses. The amount of toxin wasn't enough to kill the animals, but their immune systems would make antibodies to bind the toxin.

The serum that was on its way to Nome was made from the blood of these animals. While the public health board was arranging a shipment from Seattle, which would arrive in early February, a doctor in Anchorage found a supply—just 300,000 units, enough to keep the outbreak under control until the shipment of

1.1 million units could arrive. He wrapped it in a quilt and handed it to the conductor of the Anchorage-to-Nenana train.

HERO DOGS

A typical day's work for a musher delivering mail was about twenty or thirty miles. But long-distance dogsled racing was also a sport, and some mushers were exceptionally good at it. Leonhard Seppala was a three-time winner of the All-Alaska Sweepstakes, covering 400 miles in four days, so he was chosen for the last leg of the grueling trip.

Another accomplished musher, "Wild Bill" Shannon, picked up the quilt-wrapped bundle at the railway station and headed out on the trail. Temperatures were as low as −61° Fahrenheit, and Shannon sometimes ran behind the sled to stay warm. He developed hypothermia and frostbite on his face before handing off the package to the next musher.

Twenty teams were involved in the relay. When the mushers stopped at road houses, they warmed the serum over a fire to keep it from freezing. On the third day, a musher showed up with two of his dogs in the sled, dead from exposure. In total, over 160 dogs participated in the relay, and four died.

The run was completed in six days, but with several near misses. Seppala missed the telegram saying that the plan had been changed from a two-musher relay to one with twenty mushers. He was on his way to what he thought was the rendezvous point when another musher, who had stopped to untangle his dogs' leads, called out to him, "The serum! The serum! I have it here!"

Later on the trail, a storm blew over a musher's sled, dumping the package into the snow. The musher dug through snowdrifts with his bare hands and finally found it.

Five and a half days after the serum left the railway station, it showed up at Dr. Welch's door. President Calvin Coolidge later presented the mushers with gold medals. A statue in New York's Central Park honors Balto, the dog who led the last leg.

Five or six deaths were recorded in the outbreak, depending on the account, although Dr. Welch speculated that there could be up to 100 more among Alaska Natives who couldn't or didn't visit the hospital. The outbreak was fully contained with the larger shipment of serum, delivered later that month by many of the same mushers and teams.

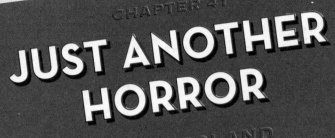

CHAPTER 41

JUST ANOTHER HORROR

TYPHUS: POLAND
1945

AS IF THE STARVATION AND TORTURE WEREN'T ENOUGH, CONCENTRATION CAMPS ALSO TENDED TO BE HOTBEDS OF TYPHUS.

DEATH TOLL: Unknown; starvation and disease, combined, were responsible for 20–30 million deaths during World War II

CAUSED BY: Bacteria in the genus *Rickettsia*, carried by the bite of body lice

NOTEWORTHY SYMPTOMS: Fever, rash, delirium

FATALITY RATE: Up to 40 percent without treatment

THREAT LEVEL TODAY: Typhus still kills 200,000 people each year, but can be controlled by washing yourself and your clothes regularly.

NOTABLE FACT: Anne Frank and her sister died of typhus shortly before their concentration camp was liberated.

The disease nicknamed "war fever" was no stranger to battle-fields and crowded bunkers, but it took an extra sinister turn in Nazi-controlled Poland. The Germans encouraged typhus epidemics among the Jews, and used the disease as an excuse to commit further atrocities. But this war would prove to be typhus's last stand.

In hundreds of cities across Nazi-occupied Poland, Germans rounded up Jews and crammed them into ghettos. Among the flimsy reasons for why they had to do this, a major one was disease. Jewish areas were full of typhus, they said, so they needed to make sure anybody infected stayed inside and couldn't get out. The ghettos were thus similar to the houses of victims of the Great Plague of London. The inhabitants were shut up and left to die, except here the deaths were not a family at a time, but thousands together.

The Germans carted in bricks and mortar, and built a wall around each ghetto. Food was supplied, but only about 300 calories per day—basically starvation rations. Anybody caught leaving the ghetto would be shot. Inside, the epidemic raged. Typhus loves crowded, filthy places in wintertime. It's transmitted by body lice, which make their home in folds of clothing. If you strap a few layers of wool to your body, and don't take them off until spring, you have created a perfect habitat for lice. The tiny insects lay their eggs in your clothes, enjoying the microclimate created by your body's heat and humidity. When they get hungry, they venture to the skin's surface for a snack of blood.

Head lice and body lice are related species, but occupy different territory as if by agreement. Head lice gross out parents and school nurses, but that's the limit of their harm. Body lice are picky about temperature, and find heads too warm. And body lice are the only ones that spread the dreaded typhus.

When the ghettos were sealed, somebody—maybe many somebodies—had the typhus germ in their body. Before long, somebody else had it too.

A PLAYGROUND FOR TYPHUS

Typhus epidemics are a cold-climate phenomenon. People bundle up in layers of clothing, giving the lice plenty of places to snuggle up. Washing your clothes once a week is enough to disrupt the louse's life cycle, but that doesn't mean avoiding typhus was always easy. Before the days of central heating and running water, taking off your clothes to bathe was not a fun winter activity. People might not bother undressing all winter. If your village was mostly free of typhus, you were dirty, but otherwise fine.

But typhus really thrives in wars and jails and, yes, concentration camps. If you're packed onto a train with starving refugees, you won't be taking a shower anytime soon, and you don't have an extra set of clothes to change into. If you live in a war-torn village, you might not have any fuel to heat water for a bath, or even to thaw your frozen water pipes in the first place. Lice thrive in these conditions. Hug your kids, and lice can crawl from you to them, or vice versa. Bump a dirty bunk bed, and lice will be among the detritus that falls from the upper level to the lower. And when you finally fall sick from typhus, the lice will make their exodus. They are sensitive to heat, and do not like being on a feverish person. They are also sensitive to cold, so any remaining lice will leave you when you die.

The infected louse finds its way to the next person, but it does not inject the germ into the person's bloodstream. Its mouth is clean, but as it eats it defecates. The bite itches, so you scratch, and rub the typhus-infected feces into the tiny wound.

The initial symptoms of typhus are a fever and headache, followed by a rash of little red spots on the chest and arms. In the later stages a delirium develops, causing hallucinations and confusion. Typhus patients may lose their sight or hearing or memory, either temporarily or sometimes for good. People in the throes of the disease may flail or grab, and a state-of-the-art typhus ward at that time would have leather straps for holding patients in bed. Suicides were not unheard of: patients would throw themselves out of windows or run out into the street.

THE BEGINNING OF THE END

As the Nazis came to power, typhus was a fresh memory, especially in Poland. An epidemic in Serbia in 1914 killed 150,000 people. Another spread across Russia in 1920, killing an estimated 3 million. Although the worst was over, soldiers and refugees had brought the germ home with them. Even after a person recovers from typhus, the bacterium still lives inside a few cells and can pop out years later, giving it a way to emerge and start new epidemics.

Even as the Germans sealed Jews into ghettos, they were terrified of the disease. Between the world wars, scientists in a few places had developed vaccines against typhus. One of these labs was Rudolf Weigl's, in Lviv, Poland (now Ukraine). Weigl knew that epidemic typhus couldn't be kept alive in convenient animals like guinea pigs, so he transferred it painstakingly from louse to louse. Since an infected louse has intestines full of the germ (to produce those infectious feces), Weigl or a member of his staff would slice a louse open with a tiny scalpel, remove the intestines, and grind them into a slurry. Later, a technician looking through a microscope would hold a fresh louse in tweezers and inject the slurry into its anus. The vaccine was made this way, with thousands of lice needed for each person vaccinated. A good dissector could do 300 louse intestines per hour. Many dissectors were needed, and many more feeders. Lice need human blood to survive. Weigl employed an army of feeders to provide their blood to lice.

Weigl disagreed with the Nazis, but agreed to produce the vaccine for them. He turned his lab into a sanctuary for Poles who would otherwise be shipped off to concentration camps: professors, musicians, and other "intelligentsia." Any officer who stopped them in the street would see their work pass, stamped "Army High Command" and "Instutite for Typhus and Viral Research" to indicate that their work was critical for defense. "Weigl was a bit like Oskar Schindler" (who was portrayed in the movie *Schindler's List*), said Arthur Allen in his book *The Fantastic Laboratory of Dr. Weigl*. Except that to get on Weigl's list, you had to strap tiny cages of lice to your legs.

Weigl and his staff sent vaccine to the Germans, probably saving thousands of lives on the front. But they also smuggled over 30,000 doses out of the lab and into ghettos, sometimes under the guise of human experiments, sometimes as doses sold on the black market, but mostly as off-the-books bulk deliveries to the Polish Institute of Hygiene.

One of Weigl's staff, a Jew named Ludwik Fleck, ended up in the Buchenwald concentration camp, where an SS doctor was running a lab dedicated to coming up with its own typhus vaccine. The prisoners were given a protocol from the Pasteur Institute in France that called for growing the germs in rabbit lungs. When it didn't work, the boss agreed to hide that fact to pad his own resume, and the lab sent useless doses of vaccine to the front. Meanwhile, Fleck figured out how to finally get the germ to grow in rabbit lungs. He and his staff made real doses of vaccine, to give to other prisoners in the camp and to send as a sample anytime the higher-ups questioned if there was something up with such-and-such vaccine lot.

Prisoners at this camp, and others, suffered terribly from typhus—sometimes given to them on purpose as a medical experiment—alongside all the other horrors, including starvation and surprise executions. "De-lousing" was part of the routine, requiring prisoners to strip in the freezing cold and take scalding-hot showers while their clothes were either steamed or treated with chemicals. At some camps, the clothes were confiscated and the "showers" turned out to be gas chambers.

When the Allies finally liberated concentration camps—including Buchenwald—they dusted prisoners with a new insecticidal powder called DDT. Both sides now had typhus vaccines, but it was the insecticides that put an end to the association of lice with war. Soldiers were given DDT powder to sprinkle in their sleeping bags and on their clothes. Although it got a nasty reputation later as a possible carcinogen and a definite environmental disaster, DDT was safe for short-term use and definitely preferable to catching typhus.

CHAPTER 42

THE BEGINNING OF THE END FOR POLIO

POLIO: USA

1952

A DISEASE THAT ATTACKS HEALTHY CHILDREN SEEMINGLY WITHOUT REASON AND CAUSES PARALYSIS, POSSIBLY CRIPPLING THEM FOR LIFE; IN 1952 POLIO BECAME EVERY PARENT'S WORST NIGHTMARE.

DEATH TOLL: Over 3,000 in 1952

CAUSED BY: Three strains of a virus known as poliovirus

NOTEWORTHY SYMPTOMS: Paralysis of arms, legs, and breathing muscles (in extreme cases)

FATALITY RATE: 5 percent among recognized infections

THREAT LEVEL TODAY: Low. The disease is almost eradicated.

NOTABLE FACT: Actors Mia Farrow and Alan Alda both contracted polio as children.

Polio had its biggest year in the United States in 1952. A major spike of cases meant that nearly 58,000 people, mostly children, were diagnosed with the disease. Of those, 3,000 died and 21,000 had lasting paralysis. The end of polio was still a few years away. Albert Sabin and Jonas Salk were working toward their respective vaccines in the lab. And in home after home across the country, children who had had some aches and pains, maybe a mild fever, were suddenly finding that they could not move a leg or an arm.

The disease was terrifying to many parents, because children seemed to be stricken randomly. Polio is caused by a virus—we had known that since 1909—and that virus could be spread when one person's intestinal secretions made it into somebody else's mouth. That's the same route that cholera takes. But in midcentury America, polio was striking families that had clean water and safe toilets, that scrubbed their houses, that lived in suburbs, not in slums. And that just made the disease seem even more random.

By the time this bumper crop of polio cases came along, whole hospital wards had been set aside for its young victims. If the paralysis had reached a child's breathing muscles, she could be kept alive in a primitive version of a ventilator, the coffin-like "iron lung." For those who could breathe but not walk, treatment included wrapping the patient in boiling-hot wool blankets. Nurses encouraged the children to be strong and independent with a tough love that sometimes bordered on abuse. Physical therapy helped to strengthen muscles, and eventually the children were outfitted with leg braces and crutches.

That equipment, and much of their hospital care, was paid for by a pioneer in fundraising: the National Foundation for Infantile Paralysis, now better known as the March of Dimes. Rather than solicit large donations from a few rich backers, the foundation asked people to collect dollars from their neighbors, to ask for donations in movie theaters, and to encourage children to send dimes to the White House.

The charity had been started in 1938 by Franklin Delano Roosevelt, who had contracted a rare adult case of polio in 1921, before his run for president. And like the children who left the polio wards on crutches, Roosevelt faced crushing stigma. He forced himself to stand and walk in public, and when he was president the Secret Service would block him from photographers' view when he was getting in and out of cars with assistance.

THE SNEAKY VIRUS

Not everybody who gets polio shows symptoms of it; the majority of cases fly under the radar. In the few people who do show symptoms, they are usually no worse than flu-like aches and fever. But occasionally, the virus invades the brain and spinal cord, and destroys the nerves that send signals to the muscles. That's when paralysis sets in.

The virus's journey begins at the mouth, where it's carried in by contaminated food or perhaps an unwashed hand. During its ten-day incubation period, the virus visits several different parts of the body. One of these places is the pair of tonsils in the back of the throat. While a few viruses begin multiplying there, others move down the digestive tract, riding on food, until they reach the small intestine. There, they find "Peyer's patches," small white areas involved in the immune system's surveillance of any germs carried in on food. But rather than being killed, poliovirus can invade Peyer's patches, and multiply there too.

From the patches it enters the lymph system, swelling lymph nodes throughout the body as it multiplies. And occasionally, if muscle is damaged by injury or if the virus manages to hitch a ride into the brain or spinal cord, the virus can latch on to proteins on the surface of a certain type of neuron. These neurons are the nerve cells that tell muscles when to contract. The virus goes on the attack and begins turning the neurons into factories for making more virus. Sometimes the nerve cells manage to fight back; if the virus wins, the neuron is destroyed, and a small area of muscle loses its ability to contract. But even cells that win the fight are damaged to a certain extent. Although they can rebuild the branches that connect to muscle, those branches are likely to be smaller and weaker than before.

With damaged neurons, children with polio are unable to move some of their muscles, or they find them weakened. Even muscles that seem to be unaffected, or that seem to recover, are often controlled by weakened, overworked neurons. The nerves will never be the same, but exercise can help to grow the muscles, helping the child to gain back some of the lost strength.

A SHIFT IN RESEARCH

Polio wasn't truly a newcomer in 1952. Although it was unknown before the nineteenth century, it may have always been with us. If this theory is true, the 1952 outbreak was only unusual because so many people were paralyzed, and that might be because of, not in spite of, the nation's newfound cleanliness.

The theory goes something like this: Poliovirus has always been around. (An ancient Egyptian carving famously shows a priest with a cane and a paralyzed leg; he's considered to be the first documented case of polio.) But we never noticed polio because most of the time, the effects are minor. Even today, 72 percent of people who are infected have no symptoms at all.

But when toilets and clean water became universal, children's immune systems no longer met the virus in the first few months after birth, when they still had their mother's antibodies coursing through their blood. They encountered the virus later in life, when it was more likely to cause paralysis rather than a mild or invisible illness.

America had an earlier, large outbreak of the disease in 1916, and at the time cats were thought to be one of the carriers. Later, suspicion shifted to flies that might be able to carry fecal matter on their tiny feet, or to swimming pools where a stray virus might survive the chlorine. In particularly bad summers, parents would sometimes forbid their children to go swimming or to socialize with other kids at movie theaters.

An early wave of polio research, funded by the group that would become the March of Dimes, attempted to figure out why polio strikes the people it does. Why children more than adults? Why boys more than girls? Why European Americans more than African Americans? Why older children more than younger ones?

The research into those questions was inconclusive. Finally, the day came when it didn't matter anymore. Several teams had been working on vaccines; Jonas Salk's team figured it out first, and the injectable Salk vaccine was licensed in 1955. Rival Albert Sabin's vaccine came later, in 1960. It carries a slightly larger risk of side effects, but can be given orally and can also prevent people from transmitting the virus to others, making it practical for mass vaccination campaigns. Those campaigns, by the way, have been wildly successful. Polio is almost extinct, today only circulating in two countries (Afghanistan and Pakistan) in the world.

CHAPTER 43

BREAKBONE FEVER

DENGUE HEMORRHAGIC FEVER: PHILIPPINES

1953

FLUID LEAKS FROM BLOOD VESSELS INTO SURROUNDING TISSUES, CAUSING INSUFFICIENT FLOW OF BLOOD TO MAJOR ORGANS AS WELL AS THE SEVERE MUSCLE AND JOINT PAIN THAT GIVES THIS DISEASE ITS OMINOUS NAME.

DEATH TOLL: Unknown

CAUSED BY: Four viruses in the *Flavivirus* genus

NOTEWORTHY SYMPTOMS: Fever; muscle and joint pain

FATALITY RATE: 1 percent for mild cases, but as high as 50 percent for severe cases that go untreated

THREAT LEVEL TODAY: Growing. Dengue sickens 96 million people each year, causing 15,000 deaths.

NOTABLE FACT: Unlike other diseases, having one of the four strains of this disease does not protect you from getting the others. In fact, it can lead to even more disastrous consequences.

E ight years after Manila saw one of the bloodiest battles of World War II, the capital of the Philippines was facing another tragedy—smaller to be sure, but terrifying just the same.

Children were showing up at hospitals severely sick, listless, and with high fevers. They also had petechiae, little red spots all over their bodies from burst capillaries, each of which leaked a little bit of blood. Often they had had a fever for days, sometimes a week or more. Maybe there was vomiting or diarrhea, or maybe they were complaining of pain all over the body. Many of these children died.

Some adults were infected too, many of them migrant workers. Adults who had lived in the area all their lives were less likely to develop the new disease—which would seem to suggest that they had some immunity, that they had seen it before. But the disease seemed to be new.

In fact, it wasn't. Later, analysis would show that the "Philippine hemorrhagic fever," like the Thai hemorrhagic fever and other, similar outbreaks happening around the same time, was caused by a virus that was familiar all over Southeast Asia: dengue virus. Normally, dengue fever is painful and exhausting but not life-threatening. It causes a high fever, often 104° Fahrenheit or more, flu-like symptoms, and in many cases serious aches and pains. The headache, muscle pain, and joint pain can be so bad that they earn the disease the name of breakbone fever.

But these kids in the Philippines were different. They bled inside their bodies and their organs failed.

WAR CHANGED EVERYTHING

World War II had disrupted everything about Southeast Asia. People who lived in the area were trying to find a normal life again, but much was changed forever.

Manila had been occupied by the Japanese and then by the Allies. The Battle for Manila had destroyed the city, flattening buildings and killing 100,000 people, mostly civilians. During the war years, people alternately moved to cities when food and jobs were scarce and evacuated in flights to safety. Japanese and Allied ships moved men and supplies from island to island, nation to nation. They brought new diseases, or they picked up old ones and took them on tour.

This was the world that birthed the twentieth-century dengue pandemic. Ships brought *Aedes aegypti* mosquitoes, an African species that colonized the Americas centuries before, to replace or live alongside native Southeast Asian species. The debris of war made plenty of places for mosquitoes to breed. No longer limited to pockets of water in jungle canopies, or its now familiar breeding spots in flower pots and old tires, mother *Aedes aegypti* mosquitoes could give their larvae good homes in the water barrels that were standing in for the destroyed water supply lines. They also had their pick of discarded war equipment and the debris of blasted-out buildings.

But even that was not enough to explain what happened. People moved, too, including military men who had no immunity to dengue and could pick it up in one country and transmit it to mosquitoes in another. After the war, people moved to new places to find jobs and steady food supplies.

The dengue virus has four types, and most areas of Southeast Asia only knew one. In the postwar period, some places were experiencing a condition called hyperendemicity: instead of one disease in residence, they had two versions living in parallel, in the same population. This would prove to be a deadly combination.

DOUBLE WHAMMY

Severe dengue, as it came to be called, seems to be most common in people who have had one type of dengue in the past, and later are hit with a second, different type.

In some diseases, previous experience with a virus is a good thing. If you've had smallpox or chickenpox once, your body remembers how to make antibodies against it and you can fight it off easily the next time. Essentially, it means you can't come down with the disease again. (This is the same idea behind vaccines: you're given just enough of a virus to make the antibodies, so you get the protection without having to suffer through the disease.)

In some cases, the immunity from one germ is enough to protect you against others that are closely related. That's why a vaccine made from cowpox can protect a person against smallpox, and why infection with tuberculosis seems to make people less prone to the related disease of leprosy.

But with dengue, something a little different happens. A person with dengue will make two types of antibodies: the neutralizing type, which helps to destroy the enemy they bind to; and a non-neutralizing type that actually helps the virus to infect cells. As long as both are active, there's no problem; the virus can still be killed. That's what will happen if you get the same strain of dengue a second time. No problem.

But a person who becomes infected with a different strain is in a different situation. The non-neutralizing antibody may become activated, but without its partner to keep it in check. In about 5 percent of people, a new set of symptoms develop that can be deadly.

Fluid leaks out of blood vessels and into the surrounding tissues. Blood may leak too, causing the person to bleed into the membranes around the brain, or in other body parts like the intestines. Needle marks from routine injections and blood draws may turn into large, ugly bruises. This is dengue hemorrhagic fever.

It can get worse, leading to dengue shock syndrome. The body, reacting to loss of blood and fluid, develops cold, clammy hands and feet. Pulse and blood pressure are weak or undetectable. The body's organs can fail from lack of blood. The mortality rate is just a few percent with good treatment, but a child who doesn't get high-quality care right away has a chance of dying that may be as high as 44 percent.

There is not yet a vaccine available for dengue, and while treatment helps there is no sure-fire cure. The changes set off by World

War II continue today: plenty of areas of the world now have *Aedes aegypti* mosquitoes, and more than one serotype of dengue virus. In some areas, severe dengue is one of the major causes of hospitalization and death among children. Even the uncomplicated versions of dengue are spreading. Florida, for example, has had several outbreaks since 2010.

The World Health Organization is working in many countries against rising numbers of dengue cases, now a serious public health concern worldwide. The postwar outbreak in the Philippines was the beginning of a worldwide pandemic that doesn't show any signs of slowing down.

CHAPTER 44

THE BRAIN-EATING AMOEBA

PRIMARY AMEBIC MENINGO-ENCEPHALITIS: AUSTRALIA

1965

WATCH YOUR NOSE IF YOU GO SWIMMING IN WARM WATER! THIS AMOEBA IS RARE, BUT CAUSES A FAST AND FATAL BRAIN INFECTION.

DEATH TOLL: 10 cases in a 15-year period

CAUSED BY: The amoeba *Naegleria fowleri*

NOTEWORTHY SYMPTOMS: Fever, runny nose, death

FATALITY RATE: Nearly 100 percent once symptoms start

THREAT LEVEL TODAY: Low. Cases are very rare.

NOTABLE FACT: Chlorine seems to be able to kill the amoebas, so most swimming pools are safe.

January is summer in South Australia. Temperatures can easily reach 100° Fahrenheit, and a popular place to cool off is the shore's seawater pools. These are built on the edge of the beach, so that waves can crash into the pool. In Port Augusta in 1961, children splashed in the pools, and most went home healthy. But one seven-year-old boy picked up an amoeba there, a tiny microbe that would travel up his nose and into his brain, killing him.

Sometime in the next week or two, he became lethargic and uninterested in playing. After two days of that, he came down with a sore throat, vomiting, and fever. His parents took him to a doctor, who gave him antibiotics. The next day, though, he was worse. He vomited more, his muscles twitched, and his neck was stiff. He went into a coma and was admitted to the local hospital. There, doctors took a sample of the fluid from around his spinal cord to see if he had meningitis. The fluid was full of pus. Immediately he was given an IV with fluids and three different antibiotics. The next day he was transferred to the children's hospital 190 miles down the coast in Adelaide, but it was too late. He died the same day.

One death like this is tragic, but then it turned out to be part of a pattern. Four years later, two girls and a man died after experiencing the exact same symptoms. The doctors looked back at medical records and found an earlier death that fit the same pattern. Meanwhile, another man and another boy had died. That made seven cases, all fatal.

CLUES FROM THE BRAIN

The doctors figured that the autopsy would show signs of the usual type of meningitis, which was caused by bacteria. What they found was shocking.

Each victim's brain was "swollen only moderately," they wrote. There was some pus in the wrinkles of the brain, indicating that white blood cells had been there fighting infection. But the part of the brain closest to the nose was red, soft, and sticky. It was completely destroyed.

Under the microscope, the doctors could see the culprit: amoebas. Not the usual invisible viruses, or tiny-but-mighty bacteria, but blobs the size of our own cells or bigger that eat bacteria and other cells for lunch. They were all over the destroyed olfactory lobes, which is the first stop for nerves carrying signals of the sense of smell. They had eaten their way through blood vessels, and then followed the little veins and arteries into other areas of the brain. (The doctors published photo after photo in their reports, to warn others about what they should look for in cases like these.)

The amoeba turned out to be a species of *Naegleria*, which normally lives in soil and doesn't bother anybody. But in a few rare cases—and we still don't know why—it can infect a person through his nose. Drinking infected water or breathing tiny droplets, like spray in the shower, won't do the trick. For *Naegleria* to infect you, you need to get the amoeba-containing water inside your nose. Maybe you snorted some seawater while you were swimming. Your nose is lined with millions of nerve cells for smelling, and a nerve runs a short distance from there to the brain. This is the highway the amoebas travel.

WORLDWIDE, BUT STILL RARE

Neither the amoeba nor its disease turned out to be unique to Australia. Soon there were seven cases in the United States, then a few in New Zealand, then more in Australia. But it took years to amass that list. From 1962 to 2014, the United States logged just 133 cases, most of them in Texas and Florida. Fifteen countries across the world have reported cases of the disease. In Pakistan, washing before prayer has been linked to cases of the amoeba disease. Religious rules don't require pushing water into the nostrils, but some worshipers do it anyway. Flushing the nose with salt water, done to relieve cold symptoms in India and across the world, has also been associated with cases. Otherwise, the disease is usually linked with swimming pools, spas, and sometimes water parks.

But you don't have to hang up your pool pass just yet. Chlorinated pools don't seem to be a problem; the amoeba comes from soil, and chlorine kills it just fine. Temperature also matters. The known cases are linked with warm water, like ponds and pools fed by hot springs, or that subtropical Australian ocean water. Cool water seems to be safe, and you can always wear a nose clip just to be sure.

Mysteries remain. The amoeba infects children far more often than adults, and men more often than women. We don't know why; maybe it's related to exposure—for example, kids are more likely than adults to play splashing and dunking games in the pool. We also don't know why it infects people in the first place. This is a microbe that scientists call "free-living." It doesn't need an animal or anyone else to act as its host; it can live its life in dirt or pond water, eating the bacteria it finds crawling or floating around. And we don't know why so many people can swim in a warm, *Naegleria*-filled pond yet only one person every couple of years comes down with the fatal illness.

Happily, the fatality rate has been dropping. A few people have survived the infection, bringing it down from 100 percent fatal to somewhere around 95 percent. The next question to answer is *why* those people survived. The disease was caught early—unlike cases that were only diagnosed at autopsy—so that's probably part of it. Doctors also sometimes tried daring therapies like cooling the body, which can slow down the course of an infection, although it's risky for the patient. Perhaps one day we'll understand this disease better, and drop that fatality rate even further.

CHAPTER 45

THE LEAK FROM COMPOUND 19

ANTHRAX: USSR

1979

WHEN PEOPLE DOWNWIND OF A GOVERNMENT FACILITY DEVELOP SYMPTOMS OF ANTHRAX POISONING AND SUBSEQUENTLY DIE, THE SOVIET GOVERNMENT SETS ABOUT COVERING ITS TRACKS.

DEATH TOLL: At least 68

CAUSED BY: The bacterium *Bacillus anthracis*

NOTEWORTHY SYMPTOMS: Fever, cough, and chest pain

FATALITY RATE: 86 percent

THREAT LEVEL TODAY: Low to medium. Natural cases of anthrax are rare in developed countries, but it is still a prime choice as a biological weapon.

NOTABLE FACT: The Soviet Union's bioweapons program began all the way back in 1928, investigating ways to weaponize typhus.

The reports began to trickle out of the Soviet Union in the autumn of 1979. They told two different stories, and both were wrong.

One account, published in a Russian dissident magazine, told of an explosion at a military base in Yekaterinburg where biological weapons were being produced. A thousand people died, said the article, because they had breathed in anthrax spores released in the accident. The government sent public health officials into the city to wash buildings with hoses and pave streets in a town that previously had all dirt roads.

Official reports denied the story. Buildings were always washed this time of year as part of the preparations for May Day, they said. Anthrax is a livestock disease, so rural areas often have minor epidemics that kill sheep and cows. The Soviet government explained that some cattle had gotten sick, and some of their meat was sold on the black market. People bought that meat, and got sick too. Sixty-four of them died.

The Soviet government found itself having to document the details of the outbreak for an international audience. Manufacturing anthrax spores as weapons would be a violation of the Biological Weapons Convention treaty signed in 1972. If the outbreak was truly from livestock, the government would be in the clear.

They pointed to livestock deaths that occurred days before people began to get sick, and traced the infection back to contamination at a plant that produced cattle feed. In presentations at scientific meetings in Washington, D.C.; Baltimore; and Cambridge, Massachusetts, Soviet public health officials flicked through slide after slide showing gory lesions in victims' intestines, agreeing with the idea that the infections began with food they had eaten. Suspiciously, they didn't bring any slides of the patients' lungs.

ANTHRAX AS A WEAPON

Why would an obscure cattle disease be at the top of governments' lists of biological weapons? From a military point of view, the bacterium that causes anthrax—*Bacillus anthracis*—is a superstar because of its spores. *B. anthracis* normally lives buried in the soil. But whenever it's starved of certain nutrients, or if it comes in contact with air, it forms spores. Spores can survive conditions that ordinary bacteria can't, and spores can also be carried through the air. Spores mean survival.

To execute this survival strategy, a single bacterial cell copies its DNA, just as it would do if it were about to split into two cells. But then the script changes. One of the copies is surrounded by a thick protective coating, creating a small packet that can survive long after the parent cell dies. Like baby Superman packed into a tiny spaceship and sent forth from his home planet, the spore is small and unassuming, but packs serious potential.

Anthrax is fairly easy to grow in the lab. With a little work, you can even get it to produce spores. But to turn it into a weapon, you need to be able to turn the spores into a very fine powder. Throw a handful of sand into the air. The grains will come crashing back down. Now drop an open bag of flour. The particles are smaller, and some of them will stay airborne a little longer. Stay in the kitchen, and burn something on the stove. The particles from the smoke are smaller still, and will hang in the air for minutes, if not hours.

"Weaponized" anthrax has been ground into powder as fine as smoke particles. A few thousand spores, puffed into the air, can cause disease in whoever breathes them in. You wouldn't have to get anyone to touch or eat them, although anthrax can also spread that way. You could just, perhaps, use a fan to blow a few grams of powdered spores over your target city.

THE INVESTIGATION
After the fall of the Soviet Union, biologist Matthew Meselson thought it might be possible to learn what really happened in Sverdlovsk more than a decade before. He put together a team of researchers and flew to Russia. His wife, Jeanne Guillemin, was the trip's anthropologist. She interviewed the victims' families and

documented the expedition in her book *Anthrax: The Investigation of a Deadly Outbreak*.

Anna Komina's story was a typical one. She had worked at a ceramics factory, and one day complained of feeling faint and dizzy, and having trouble breathing. A few days later she felt better, but then suddenly collapsed. Her adult son called the doctor, who called an ambulance. Emergency responders worked for five hours to get her blood pressure stable enough to take her to the hospital, where she died the next day. Hospital officials would not let the family take her body back for a funeral. Police guarded her coffin as it was driven to the cemetery, where she was buried in a section dedicated to anthrax cases. The death certificate read "bacterial pneumonia."

Other families had similar stories to tell. The people who died—and those who got sick but recovered—had almost all worked at the ceramics factory or nearby. Only adults died, mainly men, but no children. Although authorities said the tainted meat was sold on the black market, including at the ceramics factory, many of the victims only ate meat from state stores or from their own backyard pigs.

The team's final report told a different story. Although victims lived all over town, which fit with the tainted meat theory, their daytime locations told a different story. The ceramics factory was just downwind of the military's Compound 19. So was another military building, Compound 32. People who were in these two areas on the afternoon of April 2, 1979, were exposed to anthrax spores, as were a few residents further downwind. Remember the government's stories of anthrax breaking out in livestock? Those cases occurred at the same time as the human cases, but because veterinarians are more used to diagnosing anthrax, they detected it earlier. Several villages had anthrax outbreaks in livestock, and all of those villages sat in a line directly downwind of Compound 19. The wind was blowing southeast that day.

It only takes a tiny whiff of spores to infect a single person. Based on the number of people who got sick, Meselson and his team calculated that the amount released was less than a gram. It could have been as low as 2 milligrams. Although thousands of spores are needed to infect the average person, tests on monkeys suggest that 2 percent of the population can be infected with just nine microscopic spores.

The real cause of the outbreak emerged later. Ken Alibek, a Soviet official who was not there but says he knows the inside story, explains in his tell-all book *Biohazard* that the cause of the outbreak was a missing filter in the compound's exhaust system. A worker removed it for cleaning at the end of a shift, and left a written notice for his supervisor. The supervisor of the next shift never got the message, and turned the system back on without the filter. By the time the mistake was discovered, it was too late.

CHAPTER 46

AIDS PANIC AND PROGRESS

AIDS: USA

1980s

REPORTS OF A NEW, SEEMINGLY UNSTOPPABLE DISEASE THAT WOULD DESTROY YOUR IMMUNE SYSTEM, LEAVING YOU VULNERABLE TO A HOST OF OTHER HORRIFIC DISEASES, CAUSED WIDESPREAD PANIC IN THE UNITED STATES.

DEATH TOLL: By 1985, 12,000 deaths had been reported, out of 15,000 cases

CAUSED BY: The human immunodeficiency virus

NOTEWORTHY SYMPTOMS: A weakened immune system

FATALITY RATE: 100 percent at first; today, AIDS is not necessarily a fatal disease

THREAT LEVEL TODAY: 36.9 million people are living with HIV. Of those, 22 million do not have access to treatment.

NOTABLE FACT: The first drug to control HIV was approved in 1987. Today, there are dozens.

The first public notice that some kind of epidemic might be going on came in a government report that more often reports on how many people have the flu in a particular winter, or where there might be a few more rabies cases than usual. In June 1981 the *Morbidity and Mortality Weekly Report* announced that a rare but otherwise unremarkable lung infection was occurring in people who would normally never get it.

They were five young men, most of them previously healthy. Two were dead by the time the report came out. What were they doing with *Pneumocystis* pneumonia? Their doctors dug for clues. None of them knew each other. They all had fungal infections in their mouths, and in the past had been infected with the usually harmless cytomegalovirus. All were gay, and two admitted to having multiple recent partners. The report's writers and editors were baffled, and a note speculated whether the disease might be related to "some aspect of a homosexual lifestyle or [a] disease acquired through sexual contact." Soon gay men all over the country were turning up at hospitals with rare infections and cancers. One of these was Kaposi's sarcoma, a disease of pimple-like tumors caused by a virus.

The disease didn't get much attention from the public at first—and when it did, it was branded as a "gay plague" or "gay cancer." An early name for the disease was GRID, for gay-related immune deficiency, but that didn't stick. Soon the same infections were turning up in intravenous drug users, in people who received blood transfusions, and in hemophiliacs who depended on blood-derived clotting factors. The patients included women and children. What they had found was what is now called AIDS: the acquired immune deficiency syndrome.

Reports trickled in from all over the world. There were cases in Europe and Australia. Zambia, in southern Africa, saw a cluster of cases of Kaposi's sarcoma. Nearby, the Democratic Republic of Congo saw an increase in another rare infection, cryptococcosis. And finally, by 1984, French and U.S. scientists had both announced that they had identified the cause: a virus.

PANIC

The culprit was named the human immunodeficiency virus, or HIV. With the realization that "gay cancer" could spread from person to person, even if they weren't gay, came a public panic. A 1983 issue of *New York* magazine carried a story about how "AIDS anxiety" was transforming the city, and it carried dozens of stories demonstrating everything from reasonable fears to far-fetched panic. Medical staff in some parts of the city were reluctant to draw blood from patients who had AIDS. A police officer sopped up blood from an accident victim's head wound, and wondered if she should worry. A woman whose husband contracted AIDS suddenly found that other families were telling their children not to play with her daughter. The article wryly summarized:

"Not one of the hundreds of doctors who are studying AIDS has suggested that we are facing some twentieth-century version of the Black Death. Yet, as imaginations have become infected with fear, paranoia, and superstition, AIDS victims have been fired from their jobs, driven from their homes, and deserted by their loved ones. Any homosexual or Haitian has become an object of dread. [Some of the early AIDS cases were in Haitian immigrants.] And New York in 1983 has become a place where a woman telephones Montefiore Medical Center and asks if her children should wear gloves on the subway."

Two years later, the virus had its first celebrity death: Rock Hudson. He filmed one last television appearance with Doris Day, then flew to France for an experimental AIDS treatment. While there, he got a get-well phone call from his old Hollywood friend, President Ronald Reagan. So far, Reagan hadn't said a word about AIDS publicly. His press secretary had laughed off questions about whether the president should be concerned about the growing epidemic among gay men. Nancy Reagan even declined to call in a favor for Hudson at the French hospital where he was seeking treatment; a White House staffer wrote that "she did not feel this was something the White House should get into."

But with Hudson's death, and the announcement that he had AIDS, the tide turned. Surgeon General C. Everett Koop wrote a report on AIDS insisting that the disease be taken seriously. Ryan White, a teenager who had been refused entry to his own middle school after he contracted AIDS as a result of his treatment for hemophilia, found himself the friendly public face of the epidemic in the ensuing court battle. He met with celebrities, was interviewed on TV, and became the hero of the town where his family moved to get a fresh start. He lived long enough to see a TV movie made of his life. Shortly after his death, a law named after him promised money for AIDS services for those who may not otherwise be able to receive them.

THE VIRUS THAT CAUSES AIDS

Back in the 1980s, HIV was "the virus that causes AIDS." Today, the terminology is reversed: people with what used to be called AIDS are now more likely to be described as living with a severe HIV infection. People with HIV now live as long as people without it, if they receive treatment early and stay on it for life.

HIV is a retrovirus, which means it inserts copies of its genes into a person's DNA. Antiretroviral drugs interfere with this process, and the first drug to do so, called AZT, was approved in 1987. Some viruses stay pretty much the same over the years, and it's comparatively easy to develop vaccines and treatments for them. HIV, on the other hand, is a fast-evolving, squirrely virus, much like influenza. So far no vaccine has been able to reliably work against it; the virus changes too fast. It also can develop resistance to the drugs used against it, and soon it was evading AZT. But the virus is much more vulnerable when faced with multiple drugs. Doctors now typically prescribe a cocktail of three drugs at a time. They're expensive, but lifesaving.

The virus's quick evolution also means it has become milder over the years, not unlike what had happened with syphilis 500 years earlier. A virus that kills its victim quickly has a hard time spreading. From the germ's point of view, a better strategy is to infect its host with a more mild illness, giving the person more time and more opportunities to pass the disease on to others.

We've also made the virus's job harder with awareness of how to make sex safer, mainly by using condoms. Anti-HIV drugs are also used sooner than before, even before an infected person develops symptoms. And the drugs can also be used as prevention; for example, in people whose partners have HIV.

HIV infection is now a disease that can be brought under control, but it has a lot of lost time to make up. The number of new HIV diagnoses in the United States holds steady each year around 50,000, even though it's a preventable disease. And the situation is even worse in many parts of Africa, which is where the disease initially came from. The numbers are staggering: 25 million people are living with the virus, many without treatment; 11 million African children have lost one or both parents to AIDS. The disease should be controllable by now, but much more work is needed.

CHAPTER 47

MAD COW SPREADS TO HUMANS

TRANSMISSIBLE SPONGIFORM ENCEPHALOPATHY: ENGLAND

1996

AFTER YEARS OF HEARING AUTHORITIES SAY "MAD COW DISEASE" COULDN'T POSSIBLY SPREAD TO HUMANS—IT DID.

DEATH TOLL: 149 cases in the United Kingdom from 1996–2011

CAUSED BY: An infectious protein called a prion

NOTEWORTHY SYMPTOMS: Depression and anxiety; trouble walking; confusion; muscle spasms

FATALITY RATE: 100 percent

THREAT LEVEL TODAY: Low. After changes in laws about cattle feed, incidence of the disease plummeted.

NOTABLE FACT: This disease has been known for centuries in sheep, where it is called scrapie.

It was 1996. Scientists were supposed to have figured out all the ways that diseases can be transmitted: parasites, bacteria, viruses. DNA was no longer a complete enigma, so neither were inherited diseases. But now something very strange was going on.

Just in the past decade, cows had been coming down with a brand-new deadly illness that made them wobble on their feet, act aggressively, tremble and shake, and eventually go into a coma and die. People in England watched TV news stories that showed the cows shaking, while those same stories offered reassurances that it was extremely unlikely that any humans were in danger. But then in 1994 and 1995, three teenagers were diagnosed with a human version of this very disease.

The epidemic in cows was a brand-new thing, and the jump to humans was unprecedented. But the disease itself had a long and mysterious history in more than one species. Scientists and veterinarians—and, yes, human doctors—had been working on its puzzle for more than a hundred years. Since at least the eighteenth century, farmers and veterinarians knew about a syndrome in which sheep would lose coordination, shake uncontrollably, and scratch themselves incessantly. They would scratch against the ground, against trees, using their teeth to scratch their legs, until they ripped out chunks of wool and rubbed their skin raw. In England they called it scrapie. In France, it was *tremblante*.

Scrapie was always fatal, and never affected lambs, but only older sheep. It occurred on some farms but not others, suggesting that it was contagious. But some breeds of sheep never got it, even if they lived in the same flocks as affected sheep. So maybe it was hereditary. When that didn't seem to explain it either, veterinarians of that day suggested that it was from rams having too much sex or not enough sex, that it was triggered by other illnesses, that some types of feed could predispose sheep to it, that it was more common in sheep that had been frightened by thunder or dogs. In other words, it could be anything.

Then there was more experimentation, inspired by scientific findings about other diseases. Robert Koch had found in 1876 that the mysterious livestock disease anthrax was caused by a bacterium, and Louis Pasteur suggested the reason it kept recurring on farms is that worms brought the bacterial spores from buried animals up to the surface of the soil, where it contaminated the grass that the next generation of animals would eat.

Louis Pasteur's team managed to create a vaccine for the rabies virus, without ever being able to see the virus under the microscope. They had done their work with ground-up brain tissue. Inspired by Pasteur, scientists ground up the tissues inside different parts of sheep that had developed scrapie. An extract prepared from the brain caused scrapie if it was injected into another animal's brain. So, something in the brain was definitely contagious. The lymph nodes and digestive organs could also pass the disease on to other sheep, either inoculated into their brains or in their feed. However, the infectious agent was slow-acting. It would take months after infection, often two years or more, before the sheep would begin showing symptoms. Sheep's placentas also turned out to be infectious, giving a possible route for transmission: mother sheep eat their own placentas after birth, but other sheep in the flock may eat them too.

THE HUMAN CONNECTION

The first time a human got a scrapie-like disease was not in 1990s Britain, but in 1960s Papua New Guinea, just north of Australia. There, the disease began showing up suddenly in the Fore people. They called it *kuru*, from a word that means shivering. Men seemed to be immune, but children and women would tremble and shake. They would have trouble walking, and eventually become paralyzed, slip into a coma, and die. The illness was fatal every time. The German doctor who first saw the disease attempted to treat it, but his Fore guide told him to stop. This is sorcery, the guide explained, not sickness. None of your medicines will help.

Indeed, none did. Scientists examined the brains of people who had died of kuru, and found that under the microscope they looked like the brains of sheep with scrapie: blobs of protein surrounded by little bubbles. They looked almost like flowers, and were dubbed "florid" plaques.

Kuru, like scrapie, proved to be infectious in animal experiments. Transmission, in this case, was easier to understand: the Fore practiced a type of ritual cannibalism, in which the dead person became the funeral meal. Men were given the best meat, the muscle tissue. Women did the butchering; they and children ate the organs, including the brain. Nobody knows how kuru came to the island, but it was still a new disease when scientists started studying it. And by then, it was already in decline: the funeral meals were falling out of fashion.

Kuru bore some similarities to another human disease, Creutzfeldt-Jakob disease (CJD). Some cases are genetic, but most have no known cause. A few occur from transmission from brain to brain: in hospital equipment, for example, or in children given growth hormone made from human pituitary glands.

The culprit in all of these cases—infectious and genetic—is an unusual type of protein called a prion. Our DNA encodes instructions for creating thousands of different proteins, and we all carry the gene that makes the prion protein. Some people have a version that is a little bit unusual, and those people are more likely to come down with CJD. Others have versions that are resistant to CJD. But that's still not the whole story.

Proteins are made, per DNA's instructions, by chaining together specific chemicals called amino acids. But instead of just creating a long, unwieldy chain, the growing protein folds up on itself. The twenty types of amino acids determine the shape of the finished protein by the way they attract or repel each other, their size, and other chemical properties. Some of the amino acids can nestle closely with others; some need to be somewhere on an edge where they have plenty of room to themselves. Because of these properties, each string of amino acids gravitates to a specific shape. Once in the right shape, the protein can do its job in the cell. Some proteins make up the cell's structure; others are enzymes that slice or splice other chemicals, and so on.

But what if a protein doesn't fold correctly? Imagine that a protein, in folding, is supposed to insert "tab A" into "slot B." But there is a configuration where tab A is sticking out in the wrong direction, nowhere near slot B. Tab A bumps into another protein, just in the process of being folded, and occupies its neighbor's slot B. That neighbor ends up with the same problem, and disrupts another protein, and so on until great chains of the protein have built up inside the cell. This, we think, is what happens in CJD and mad cow disease. The initial misfolded protein can come from an infected animal, or it can be made by the brain cells themselves. So a prion is just a protein all by itself—not part of a living creature like a bacterium, or an arguably living, complex particle like a virus. It's just a single chain of amino acids in a dangerous shape.

That explains how the disease can be both inherited and transmitted. Many mysteries still remain: Where do the unexplained cases of CJD come from? Why did only a few people ever come down with "variant CJD," as the human version of mad cow was called? And how did people catch it by eating beef (which scientists agree must have happened) even though we've known for centuries that the meat from scrapie-affected sheep is safe to eat?

The other big question—where mad cow disease came from in the first place—has a likely answer. The British epidemic among cows probably came from an ingredient in their feed called "meat and bone meal." That's a protein supplement made from otherwise discarded meat, including the carcasses of sheep affected by scrapie. Meat and bone meal was not new, but the processing techniques changed around 1981. Prions are harder to "kill" than bacteria or viruses, and they were able to survive the newer technique.

The disease takes years before it starts showing symptoms, so the first cows weren't recognized as "mad" until 1985 at the earliest.

By the time the British government banned meat and bone meal from animal feed in 1988, cattle had been eating it for seven years. Assuming a four-year incubation period, they figured that cases in animals should start declining around 1992—which is exactly what happened. The disease then incubated for years in people who had eaten infected meat, so cases in humans weren't discovered until the mid-1990s. By the year 2000, animal cases had fallen from a peak of thousands per month to barely 100, and they are still falling.

CHAPTER 48

THE LOCKER ROOM MENACE

MRSA: LOS ANGELES

2002

A RESISTANT BACTERIA THAT CANNOT BE KILLED BY ORDINARY MEANS AND CAUSES PUS-FILLED BOILS THAT ROT AWAY FLESH—A MENACE TO BE SURE.

DEATH TOLL: Over 11,000 per year, according to 2011 data from the CDC

CAUSED BY: A methicillin-resistant version of the bacterium *Staphylococcus aureus*

NOTEWORTHY SYMPTOMS: Pus-filled boils on the skin; fever

FATALITY RATE: 15 percent or more, in severe cases

THREAT LEVEL TODAY: Although rare, MRSA has become more common than it was and can be difficult to treat once an infection begins.

NOTABLE FACT: Other types of resistant bacteria exist, and are becoming more common. They include *Clostridium difficile*, carbapenem-resistant enterobacteriaceae (CRE), and a cephalosporin-resistant strain of the bacterium that causes gonorrhea.

In the fall of 2002, a football player at the University of Southern California (USC) sought treatment for a pimple on his elbow. It was unusually painful, and he was running a low fever, barely 100° Fahrenheit.

It was a good thing he showed up at the hospital. Doctors performed surgery that day, and found that his MRSA infection had taken the form of necrotizing fasciitis, the infamous "flesh eating" bacterial infection.

In necrotizing fasciitis, bacteria don't actually "eat" flesh. They secrete toxins that destroy connective tissue, which begins to rot inside the body. Without surgery to remove the dead tissue, death or the need for amputation can result. And because the damage is the result of a thriving and growing population of bacteria, the infection will continue to spread, often in spite of treatment. The USC football player endured multiple surgeries in attempts to save his arm, and eventually needed skin grafts to cover the wounds that were left. A second player on the same team was hospitalized with an abscess on his leg. He too required surgeries, not to remove dead tissue but to drain out pockets of pus inside his leg.

Those were the only serious cases documented that year. But shortly after the 2003 season began, seventeen of the 107 players developed infections serious enough to require surgery. DNA tests showed that all of the players' infections were from the same strain of MRSA, meaning they had probably all gotten it from the same place. The rules about using antibacterial soap and avoiding the whirlpool tub with open wounds, put in place after the 2002 cases, clearly weren't enough to prevent the spread of infection. Team officials, stumped, called in the county health department to investigate.

NOT A PIMPLE

MRSA is methicillin-resistant *Staphylococcus aureus*, a version of a bacterium that normally lives harmlessly on human skin. About a third of us carry *S. aureus* in our noses; 2 percent of us have the version that is resistant to many antibiotic drugs, including methicillin. The first sign of a MRSA infection may look like a pimple, or some redness on the skin. It may look so innocent that the person doesn't even think to consult a doctor—until it gets worse.

A boil often develops, a swollen area that festers with pus. The boils look horrific and sometimes people chalk these up to "spider bites." MRSA, however, is a more realistic diagnosis for many of the wounds blamed on spiders. And the MRSA infections can move fast, causing serious complications and even death.

At first, MRSA was associated with hospitals. After all, hospitals are a common place for germs and drugs to meet. A stray germ that survives cleaning can hang around, being passed from place to place, for example on unwashed hands. Hospital-acquired MRSA is a tragedy, but it's somewhat understandable how it happens.

Then doctors began noticing patients arriving at the hospital who already had MRSA. The first published reports of these infections were met with skepticism; surely somebody in the outbreak had picked up the germ at a hospital. But the new strain had different DNA than the hospital kind, and a different repertoire of antibiotics it could survive. After many outbreaks, the scientific community had to admit that the germ was living wild and free, being passed from person to person with no hospital in sight, possibly hitching rides on shared towels or surfaces. Later, it was found in the noses of pigs on farms, where antibiotics are routinely included in their feed.

NEW RULES

MRSA is still under-appreciated, but coaches are starting to get a better handle on how to prevent the infection from plaguing a team. Contact sports like football and wrestling are particularly good at spreading skin bacteria, and those bacteria have plenty of chances to get past the skin when players get turf burns or other minor injuries.

Five players on Washington's NFL team came down with the infection in 2006, which ended defensive lineman Brandon Noble's career. Their locker room got "nuked," as Noble put it. Owners disinfected the building, swapped shared benches for individual stools, and replaced the whirlpool tub with a $17,000 model that boasted a bacteria-killing filter.

The USC football team had a smaller budget, but was eventually able to eradicate its outbreak too. After the 2002 cases, players were told not to share personal equipment, and banned from the whirlpool tub if they had any open wounds.

The following year, when the outbreak reappeared at USC, trainers and team doctors started an education campaign in hopes players would be hypervigilant about hygiene. They required players to shower immediately after games, required that open wounds be covered, and prohibited players from taking naps on piles of used towels. Players continued to get infections, and then the epidemiologists actually watched one of the football games. Although players understood they shouldn't share towels in the locker rooms, they were sharing them out on the field. Coaches ordered disposable towels.

That doesn't mean MRSA is defeated. It still pops up in NFL teams: two players for the Tampa Bay Buccaneers suffered infections bad enough in 2013 to end their careers. "It's not at all clear that teams treat . . . prevention as a routine thing they should be doing," writes science journalist Maryn McKenna, "and because of that, every athlete's infection seems like a random tragedy, instead of an avoidable mistake."

CHAPTER 49

THE SECRET EPIDEMIC

SARS: HONG KONG

2003

A DEADLY AND EXTREMELY CONTAGIOUS DISEASE BEGAN TO SPREAD IN CHINA— BUT AT FIRST, THE GOVERNMENT DIDN'T WANT ANYBODY TO KNOW ABOUT IT.

DEATH TOLL: 8,000 people in 6 months

CAUSED BY: The SARS coronavirus

NOTEWORTHY SYMPTOMS: Fever, flu-like symptoms, and pneumonia

FATALITY RATE: 10 percent

THREAT LEVEL TODAY: Low. SARS has not been seen since 2004.

NOTABLE FACT: Most of the worldwide spread can be traced to one patient who stayed in a hotel with international travelers.

Cell phones were buzzing across China's Guangdong province. Text messages carried rumors of a new, deadly disease that the government didn't want anybody to know about. The texts ricocheted across the newly popular SMS network as people forwarded messages to family and friends. Some suggested that boiling vinegar would prevent disease by purifying the air. Others endorsed over-the-counter antibiotics or a traditional medicine called *ban lan gen*. The advice may have been wishful thinking, but the secret epidemic was real, and it was SARS.

Four people, two of them chefs, had checked into hospitals with fever and coughs that did not respond to normal treatment. In their wake, at least seventeen health care workers came down with the same disease. That was in December 2002. In January 2003, as rumors were flying, the province sent public health officials to one of the affected hospitals to investigate, and one of the officials fell ill and had to be admitted.

In February, two local newspapers ran stories about a "mysterious illness." China's government began sending notices to the media that they were not to cover the epidemic. Hong Kong journalist Thomas Abraham writes in his book *Twenty-First Century Plague* that news outlets dodged the ever-increasing restrictions by reporting indirectly. Instead of saying that a disease was spreading, they said that rumors were spreading. Instead of suggesting that people take precautions, they reported on high demand for vinegar and *ban lan gen*. One article in the *Heyuan Daily* managed to report the symptoms of the disease, the pattern of its spread, and the fact that government officials were both investigating the outbreak and withholding information about it, under the headline "Epidemic Is Only a Rumor."

FACEMASKS EVERYWHERE

The symptoms of SARS (severe acute respiratory syndrome) are much like those of the common cold. The affected person has a fever, followed by respiratory symptoms like coughing, wheezing, or shortness of breath. At this point the disease is highly contagious, but people may not realize they have anything worse than a cold or flu. The disease progresses to pneumonia, and many people with SARS ended up unable to breathe. It was fatal in about 10 percent of cases, but older adults had the worst prognosis: half of patients over the age of fifty died.

The disease also spread like the common cold: through droplets from coughs and sneezes, through close personal contact, and through objects that touched the mouth or nose, like tissues and eating utensils.

Once word of the outbreak got around to hospital workers, they began using precautions—gloves, facemasks, and sometimes full-body suits—with any patients that might have the new virus. But it's hard to take a mask off cleanly every single time, when the outside might be covered in infectious particles from a SARS super-spreader. Some people only infected one or two others, but the super-spreaders left piles of corpses in their wake. Interviews with infected people and their families revealed that sometimes dozens had been in contact with the same person at the same time. One man managed to infect twenty-five health care workers, twenty fellow patients, and seventeen people he met outside the hospital.

It was during the SARS epidemic that the now-popular Asian trend of wearing facemasks in public caught on. The facemasks had come out before, during the 1918 flu and after a 1923 earthquake and fire that put ashes into the air. Now, businesses began to require their employees to wear masks at work.

In February, around the time the World Health Organization was starting to suspect that Guangdong might be harboring an epidemic of bird flu, a professor and his wife traveled from Guangdong to Hong Kong for their nephew's wedding. They stayed on the ninth floor of the Metropole Hotel, but the man fell sick and checked into the local hospital the next day. This is how the epidemic went global.

Other guests on the ninth floor included an elderly couple from Toronto, a Chinese-American businessman who was on his way to Vietnam, and tourists from Shanghai—to name just a few. From that hotel, guests carried the SARS virus to parts of the world it had never seen before. One took it to a local hospital, where it spread to an apartment building called the Amoy Gardens. The apartment residents were quarantined when more than 200 of them came down with the disease.

SOLVING THE MYSTERY

As people traveled into and out of Hong Kong and other epidemic areas, the disease spread further. On several occasions, people came down with symptoms of SARS while a plane was in the air. The United States issued its first-ever travel advisory, which it hadn't done even when there was bubonic plague in India a decade before. A retrospective from the U.S. Centers for Disease Control and Prevention summed it up: "Fragile business alliances, trade, and travel were instantly in jeopardy as people across multiple continents waited for public health scientists to solve the mystery."

By the end of March, scientists had found the virus. By the end of April, they knew the sequence of its genes. With that information, a test for the virus was possible. Health care workers around the world were on the alert for people with symptoms of the disease, and they stood with high-quality facemasks at the ready.

With efforts like these, and cooperation from health departments worldwide, the disease could be brought under control. Not with a vaccine or a cure, because there was none, but by isolating sick people and protecting hospital workers. By July, the epidemic was over. Over 8,000 people in twenty-six countries had gotten the disease, and 774 had died. The Chinese government apologized for withholding information in the beginning, when better communication could have stopped the outbreak sooner.

SARS cases are now gone from the wild, but public health officials still worry about the potential for a fatal, highly contagious coronavirus to star in another epidemic. Across the world, in Saudi Arabia, a new virus appeared a decade later. Called MERS, for Middle East respiratory syndrome, it seems to have come from camels. So far it hasn't become a world traveler like SARS. Let's hope it stays that way.

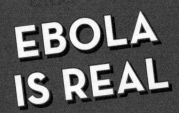

EBOLA IS REAL

THE MUCH-FEARED DISEASE SHOWED THAT ITS EARLIER DEADLY OUTBREAKS WERE JUST PRACTICE RUNS. THIS EPIDEMIC DEVASTATED MANY COMMUNITIES IN WEST AFRICA.

DEATH TOLL: At least 11,000

CAUSED BY: The virus *Zaire ebolavirus*

NOTEWORTHY SYMPTOMS: Fever, vomiting, hiccups, and sometimes bleeding from multiple body parts

FATALITY RATE: 70 percent

THREAT LEVEL TODAY: Unknown. Ebola tends to reappear unpredictably.

NOTABLE FACT: Even though the outbreak is over, scientists are learning new things about it: for example, Ebola survivors often have pockets of virus living in their eyes or other body parts.

The first case occurred in December, but nobody realized what it was until the following March. A two-year-old boy from a small village in Guinea came down with a fever, vomiting, and diarrhea. His pregnant mother took him, and his older sister, to stay with their grandmother. Within weeks, all were dead.

As the outbreak grew, its deaths were a tragedy but not an international emergency—not even a medical mystery. The symptoms matched cholera, and so the local doctors notified the health department that a cholera epidemic might be brewing. More patients died, both in the child's village and in others nearby. Some of the symptoms didn't match up to cholera, doctors noticed: sometimes there would be nosebleeds and often a high fever. Could some of the patients have malaria? Was the bleeding perhaps a sign of Lassa fever, an occasionally fatal disease transmitted by rats?

Hiccups were what gave it away. By that time, months after the first case, Doctors Without Borders was trying to figure out what was so fatal in these few villages in Guinea. The epidemiologist who read the report knew that hiccups were (for reasons we still don't understand) a symptom of hemorrhagic fevers. That could mean Lassa, a disease that kills maybe 1 percent of people infected, or Ebola. Ebola wasn't a likely suspect at first because it had never been seen in this area before. Officials in Guinea didn't even have the means to test for Ebola virus, so eventually they sent blood samples to France and nearby Senegal. The results came back positive: Not Lassa. Not malaria. Ebola.

PROTECT YOUR FAMILY, PROTECT YOUR COMMUNITY

Until that point in history, Ebola outbreaks had always been terrifying but brief. Doctors Without Borders sent aid teams immediately; the World Health Organization announced the outbreak, and the local governments activated emergency committees. Workers swooped in with protective suits, setting up field hospitals and isolating the sick. Families were not allowed to be near their loved ones, nor to take bodies home for traditional funerals, in which people would grieve as they washed and touched the body. Instead, health workers would zip the dead person into a body bag and bury it. Absolutely no touching was allowed.

The quick response meant that some villages hadn't gotten the message about the Ebola epidemic before the teams arrived. From their point of view, foreigners came in huge numbers, took people with what looked like mild illnesses and checked them into what the workers claimed was a hospital, and then whisked away nearly every one of those people in a body bag. Rumors spread that there was no such thing as Ebola and that the foreigners were running a horrific organ-harvesting operation.

Death tolls climbed higher and higher. By June, 300 people had died. By September, 3,000 had died and the number was climbing. A trio of Liberian music artists wrote a song that played on radios across the region: "Ebola Is Real." More and more people understood that the hospitals were a place to get help, that hiding a patient at home was just putting others at risk. "Protect your family, protect your community," the singers crooned. The World Health Organization issued a protocol for "safe and dignified" burials. Pages describing how to handle the body were sandwiched between others describing how to greet the family (in your street clothes) and how to tailor the procedure to include prayers and religious rituals—Christian, Muslim, or otherwise.

Ebola sufferers were treated in isolation units surrounded by a double fence so that families could see their loved ones, but couldn't reach through to touch. The doctors and health workers would put on white or yellow "space suits," complete with gloves, mask, and boots, before going in to see patients. They would make notes on paper, then shout the contents of the note to somebody on the other side of the fence. The notes would later be burned, along with the suits, which cost $80 each. Even construction workers in the area—putting up a roof, say, to shade patients from the sun—had to work in the suits despite the broiling heat.

When the workers undressed, they would do it in pairs, each watching the other to make sure there was no possibility that they were accidentally touching a bit of contaminated blood or vomit from the outside of the suit. Despite precautions, some workers got sick anyway. Liberia's top Ebola doctor was one of them. Two Americans working with a humanitarian group came down with the disease and were flown to a hospital in the United States, news vehicles chasing their ambulance down the highway and tabloids screaming about the possibility of an American epidemic. But with careful isolation of the sick, Ebola doesn't hop from person to person so easily. The few Ebola patients in the United States and other high-income countries did not spark outbreaks.

DEEP IN THE FOREST

What's really so mysterious about Ebola isn't how it appears, but how it *disappears*, traveling thousands of miles with no one the wiser. When the 2014 epidemic broke out, experts looked around for the nearest possible cache of virus. Twenty years earlier, the Taï Forest, 500 miles away, had seen an Ebola outbreak among chimpanzees that infected and killed a researcher who did an autopsy on one of the dead apes. But tests of the 2014 Ebola virus showed it wasn't related to that strain. It was, instead, the same species of virus as the one last seen in 2009 in the Democratic Republic of Congo, 2,400 miles away.

It would be difficult, but not impossible, for a person to have brought Ebola to town. He would have to fly into a nearby city, and then endure at least a twelve-hour bus ride to get to the village where the outbreak started. That's unlikely for someone who would be feverish and beset with vomiting and diarrhea. Instead, the culprit may have been a bat.

Nobody has yet found the smoking gun of a bat with an Ebola infection. But studies in various parts of Africa have found bats, including fruit bats, with antibodies showing they had probably been exposed to the virus sometime in the past. Fruit bats are big and meaty, so they're popular among hunters and in many places can be bought at markets to take home and cook. When Ebola struck villages in Guinea, scientists began to track down the first cases, eventually arriving at that of the two-year-old and his family. Those first cases didn't report hunting or eating fruit bats, but near the boy's home there was something worth looking at. A tree.

Just fifty yards from the boy's house was a large hollow tree. Children would play in and around it, locals told researchers. That tree was home to Angolan free-tailed bats, a snack-sized species that the kids would sometimes catch and eat. By the time the researchers got there, the tree had burned—whether deliberately or not, they did not say. (When it caught fire, there was a "rain of bats," the neighbors said.)

That tree may have been the source of the deadliest Ebola outbreak in history. Over a year and a half, more than 11,000 people died. Eventually the health teams' efforts succeeded. Sick people went to hospitals and stayed away from others; workers tracked down everyone who had had contact with sick people, and monitored them too. Traditional funerals gave way to prayers over body bags.

But the outbreak had lasting effects. While health clinics were crammed full of patients with Ebola, nobody wanted to come in for a checkup or to bring their kids in to get their shots. People, warned away from touching anybody who might be sick, refused to help neighbors who, say, collapsed due to heart attacks.

Some villages now stand empty. Families were torn apart: more than 3,000 children lost one or both parents to the epidemic. Those children, and people who survived the disease, face serious stigma.

One Ebola survivor, pregnant when she was released from the treatment center, told a reporter that nobody would help her when she was in labor. Her mother, a midwife, had died of the disease. The pregnant woman staggered out of her house and found herself in the middle of a crowd of women, who formed a barrier with their bodies to give her privacy while she gave birth. No one, though, would touch her or her premature baby. Her son died shortly after birth. Would help have saved him? She didn't know.

Scientists are still learning about Ebola virus disease, even after the epidemic has run its course. It turns out that even after a person has recovered, the virus can hide in parts of the body: the uterus, in pregnant women; the eyes, in many survivors. It can hide in the testicles for weeks or perhaps months, meaning that men who survive the disease may be able to pass the virus to partners sexually.

It may seem startling that, with all modern science and medicine have to offer, an epidemic can still take us by surprise. The high death rates and abandoned villages of 2014 West Africa aren't very different from what Europe must have looked like in the days of the Black Death; not very different from Squanto's hometown in illness-stricken Massachusetts.

There is still no cure for Ebola, and no reliable vaccine. It's hard to test vaccines and treatments when the disease they treat has been—if only temporarily—stamped out. Ebola will probably return. In the meantime, other diseases are bubbling under the surface that might find a way of exploding into international news.

We are lucky to have figured out the value of public health organizations that monitor new diseases as they emerge—as did the doctors who spotted Ebola back when it had claimed only a few dozen victims. We are lucky to have antibiotics and deworming medications that are effective most of the time. But it's a constant fight. Antimicrobials have stopped working against some strains of bacteria and parasites, so we need to come up with new ones and we need to take better care of the ones we have. Smallpox has been eradicated, but other diseases that stand on the brink of extinction—guinea worm and polio, for example—have outlived deadline after deadline. Doctors and scientists are doing their best, but we can never assume that we have somehow vanquished disease.

FURTHER READING

World Takeover: Malaria, Africa, 10,000 B.C.E.
McCann, James. *The Historical Ecology of Malaria in Ethiopia: Deposing the Spirits*. 2015. Athens: Ohio University Press.

Schlagenhauf, Patricia. "Malaria: From Prehistory to Present." *Infectious Disease Clinics of North America* 18, no. 2 (2004): 189–205. http://dx.doi.org/doi:10.1016/j.idc.2004.01.002.

Shah, Sonia. *The Fever: How Malaria Has Ruled Humankind for 500,000 Years*. 2010. New York: Sarah Crichton Books/Farrar, Straus, and Giroux.

The Fiery Serpent: Guinea Worm, Red Sea, 1495 B.C.E.
Hunter, John M. "An Introduction to Guinea Worm on the Eve of Its Departure: Dracunculiasis Transmission, Health Effects, Ecology and Control." *Social Science & Medicine* 43, no. 9 (1996): 1399–425. http://dx.doi.org/doi:10.1016/0277-9536(96)00043-3.

Küchenmeister, Friedrich. *On Animal and Vegetable Parasites of the Human Body: A Manual of Their Natural History, Diagnosis, and Treatment*. 1857. London: Printed for the Sydenham Society.

The Holy Bible King James Version. 1611. Cambridge, England: Cambridge University Press.

The Plague of Athens: Unknown Disease, Athens, 430 B.C.E.
Cunha, Burke A. "The Cause of the Plague of Athens: Plague, Typhoid, Typhus, Smallpox, or Measles?" *Infectious Disease Clinics of North America* 18, no. 1 (2004): 29–43. http://dx.doi.org/doi:10.1016/S0891-5520(03)00100-4.

Kazanjian, Powel. "Ebola in Antiquity?" *Clinical Infectious Diseases* 61, no. 6 (2015): 963–68. http://dx.doi.org/doi:10.1093/cid/civ418.

Papagrigorakis, Manolis J., et al. "DNA Examination of Ancient Dental Pulp Incriminates Typhoid Fever As a Probable Cause of the Plague of Athens." *International Journal of Infectious Diseases* 10, no. 3 (2006): 206–14. doi.org/10.1016/j.ijid .2005.09.001.

Thucydides, *History of the Pelopponesian War,* trans. Richard Crawley. 1920. London: Dent.

Galen's Plague: Smallpox, Rome, c.e. 165

Littman, R.J., and M.L. Littman. "Galen and the Antonine Plague." *American Journal of Philology* 94, no. 3 (1973): 243. http://dx.doi.org/doi:10.2307/293979.

Temkin, Owsei. *Galenism; Rise and Decline of a Medical Philosophy*. 1973. Ithaca, NY: Cornell University Press.

The Plague of Justinian: Bubonic Plague, Constantinople, c.e. 542

Procopius, *History of the Wars,* trans. H.B. Dewing. 1914. London: William Heinemann.

Rosen, William. *Justinian's Flea: Plague, Empire, and the Birth of Europe*. 2007. New York: Viking.

A Vicious Cycle: Smallpox, Japan, c.e. 735

Farris, William Wayne. *Population, Disease, and Land in Early Japan, 645–900*. 1995. Harvard University Asia Center.

Snodgrass, Mary Ellen. *World Epidemics: A Cultural Chronology of Disease from Prehistory to the Era of SARS*. 2003. Jefferson, NC: McFarland & Company.

Message from a Sacred Mountain: Smallpox, China, c. 1000

Carrell, Jennifer Lee. *The Speckled Monster*. 2003. New York: Dutton.

Hopkins, Donald R. *Princes and Peasants*. 1983. Chicago: University of Chicago Press.

Leung, Angela Ki Che. "'Variolation' and Vaccination in Late Imperial China, ca 1570–1911." 2011. *History of Vaccine Development*, 5–12. http://dx.doi.org/ doi:10.1007/978-1-4419-1339-5_2.

Needham, Joseph. *Science and Civilisation in China*. Vol 6, Biology and Biological Technology, Part IV, Medicine. 2000. Cambridge: Cambridge University Press.

Saint Anthony's Fire: Ergotism, France, 1095
Nemes, C.N. "The Medical and Surgical Treatment of the Pilgrims of the Jacobean Roads in Medieval Times." 2002. International Congress Series 1242: 31–42. doi.org/10.1016/S0531-5131(02)01096-8.

A Doomed Crusade: Scurvy, Egypt, 1249
Joinville, Jean, and Ethel Kate Bowen-Wedgwood. *The Memoirs of the Lord of Joinville*. 1906. London: J. Murray.

The Knights of Lazarus: Leprosy (Hansen's Disease), Europe, 1200s
Nesbitt, John W., and Timothy S. Miller. *Walking Corpses: Leprosy in Byzantium and the Medieval West*. 2014. Ithaca, NY: Cornell University Press.

Watts, S.J. *Epidemics and History: Disease, Power, and Imperialism*. 1997. New Haven, CT: Yale University Press.

China's Plague: Bubonic Plague, China, c. 1331
Kelly, John. *The Great Mortality*. 2005. New York: HarperCollins Publishers.

McNeill, William Hardy. *Plagues and Peoples*. 1976. Garden City, NY: Anchor Press.

Morelli, Giovanna, et al. "Yersinia Pestis Genome Sequencing Identifies Patterns of Global Phylogenetic Diversity." 2010. *Nature Genetics* 42 (12): 1140–1143. doi.org/10.1038/ng.705.

Orent, Wendy. *Plague: The Mysterious Past and Terrifying Future of the World's Most Deadly Disease*. 2004. New York: Free Press.

The Black Death: Bubonic Plague, Europe, 1348
Cantor, Norman F. *In The Wake of the Plague*. 2001. New York: Free Press.

Ziegler, Philip. *The Black Death*. 1991. Stroud, Gloucestershire: Sutton.

The Sweating Sickness: Unknown Disease, England, 1485
Hecker, J.F.C, B.G Babington, and John Caius. *The Epidemics of the Middle Ages*. 1859. London: Trübner.

Heyman, Paul, Leopold Simons, and Christel Cochez. "Were the English Sweating Sickness and the Picardy Sweat Caused by Hantaviruses?" 2014. *Viruses* 6 (1): 151–171. http://dx.doi.org/doi:10.3390/v6010151.

The First Invaders: Influenza, Hispaniola/Haiti, 1493
Guerra, Francisco. "The Earliest American Epidemic: The Influenza of 1493." 1988. *Social Science History* 12 (3): 305–325. http://dx.doi.org/doi:10.2307/1171451.

Mann, Charles C. *1493: Uncovering the New World Columbus Created*. 2011. New York: Knopf.

The French Disease: Syphilis, Italy, 1495
Quétel, Claude. *History of Syphilis*. 1990. Baltimore: Johns Hopkins University Press.

Rothman, David J., Steven Marcus, and Stephanie A Kiceluk. *Medicine and Western Civilization*. 1995. New Brunswick, NJ: Rutgers University Press.

Tampa, M., I. Sarbu, C. Matei, V. Benea, S. Georgescu. "Brief History of Syphilis." 2014. *Journal of Medicine and Life* 7 (1): 4–10.

The Dancing Plague: Mass Psychogenic Illness, Strasbourg, 1518
Waller, John. *The Dancing Plague: The Strange, True Story of an Extraordinary Illness*. 2009. Naperville, IL: Sourcebooks.

The Fall of Moctezuma: Smallpox, Tenochtitlán, 1520
Mann, Charles C. *1491: New Revelations of the Americas Before Columbus*. 2006. New York: Knopf.

The Lost Cure for Scurvy: Scurvy, Stadacona, 1536
Bown, Stephen R. *Scurvy: How a Surgeon, a Mariner, and a Gentleman Solved the Greatest Medical Mystery of the Age of Sail*. 2004. New York: Thomas Dunne Books, St. Martin's Press.

Cartier, Jacques, Henry Percival Biggar, and Ramsay Cook. *The Voyages of Jacques Cartier*. 1993. Toronto: University of Toronto Press.

The King's Evil: Scrofula, France, 1594
Bloch, Marc. *The Royal Touch*. 1973. London: Routledge & K. Paul.

Squanto's Backstory: Unknown Disease, Massachusetts, 1616
Humins, John H. "Squanto And Massasoit: A Struggle for Power." 1987. *New England Quarterly* 60 (1): 54. http://dx.doi.org/ doi:10.2307/365654.

Marr, John S., and John T. Cathey. "New Hypothesis for Cause of Epidemic Among Native Americans, New England, 1616–1619." 2010. *Emerging Infectious Diseases* 16 (2): 281–286. http:// dx.doi.org/doi:10.3201/eid1602.090276.

Morton, Thomas, and Charles Francis Adams. *New English Canaan of Thomas Morton*. 1967. New York: B. Franklin.

The First Miracle Cure: Malaria, Peru, 1630
Rocco, Fiammetta. *The Miraculous Fever Tree*. 2003. New York: HarperCollins.

The Great Plague of London: Bubonic Plague, London, 1665
Moote, A. Lloyd, and Dorothy C. Moote. *The Great Plague*. 2004. Baltimore: Johns Hopkins University Press.

Scourge of a Young Nation's Capital: Yellow Fever, Philadelphia, 1793
Jones, Absalom, Richard Allen, and Matthew Clarkson. *A Narrative of the Proceedings of the Black People, During the Late Awful Calamity in Philadelphia, in the Year 1793*. 1794. Philadelphia: Printed for the authors, by William W. Woodward, at Franklin's Head, no. 41, Chesnut-Street.

Murphy, Jim. *An American Plague*. 2003. New York: Clarion Books.

Peeing Red: Schistosomiasis, Egypt, 1799
Tanaka, H., and M. Tsuji. "From Discovery to Eradication of Schistosomiasis in Japan: 1847–1996." 1997. *International Journal for Parasitology* 27 (12): 1465–1480. http://dx.doi.org/ doi:10.1016/s0020-7519(97)00183-5.

The Romantic Disease: Tuberculosis, England, 1800s
Dubos, René J., and Jean Dubos. *The White Plague*. 1952. Boston: Little, Brown.

The Haitian Revolution: Yellow Fever, Saint-Domingue, 1802

Dubois, Laurent. *Haiti: The Aftershocks of History*. 2012. New York: Metropolitan Books.

Marr, John S., and John T. Cathey. "The 1802 Saint-Domingue Yellow Fever Epidemic and the Louisiana Purchase." 2013. *Journal of Public Health Management and Practice* 19 (1): 77–82. http://dx.doi.org/doi:10.1097/phh.0b013e318252eea8.

Birth of a Pandemic: Cholera, India, 1817
Barua, Dhiman, and William B. Greenough. 1992. *Cholera*. New York: Plenum Medical Book Co.

Childbed Fever: Uterine Infection, Vienna, 1847
Nuland, Sherwin B. *The Doctors' Plague*. 2003. New York: W.W. Norton.

Mapping Death: Cholera, London, 1854
Johnson, Steven. *The Ghost Map: The Story of London's Most Terrifying Epidemic—and How It Changed Science, Cities, and the Modern World*. 2006. New York: Riverhead Books.

Exiled on Molokai: Leprosy (Hansen's Disease), Hawaii, 1866
Tayman, John. *The Colony: The Harrowing True Story of the Exiles of Molokai*. 2006. New York: Scribner.

Beat of the Death-Drum: Measles, Fiji, 1875
Corney, Bolton G. "The Behavior of Certain Epidemic Diseases in Natives of Polynesia, With Especial Reference to the Fiji Islands." 1884. *Transactions of the Epidemiological Society of London*.

Tunnel of Anemia: Hookworm, Switzerland, 1880
Altman, Lawrence K. *Who Goes First? The Story of Self-Experimentation in Medicine*. 1998. University of California Press.

Brooker, Simon, Jeffrey Bethony, and Peter J. Hotez. "Human Hookworm Infection in the 21st Century." 2004. *Advances in Parasitology* 58: 197–288. http://dx.doi.org/doi:10.1016/s0065-308x(04)58004-1.

Rabies Loses Its Bite: Rabies, Paris, 1885
Debré, P. *Louis Pasteur*. 1998. Baltimore: Johns Hopkins University Press.

Wasik, Bill, and Monica Murphy. *Rabid: A Cultural History of the World's Most Diabolical Virus*. 2012. New York: Viking.

The Beriberi Box: Beriberi, Japan, 1884
Carpenter, Kenneth J. *Beriberi, White Rice, and Vitamin B*. 2000. Berkeley: University of California Press.

Hawk, Alan. "The Great Disease Enemy, Kak'ke (Beriberi) and the Imperial Japanese Army." 2006. *Military Medicine* 171 (4): 333–339. http://dx.doi.org/doi:10.7205/milmed.171.4.333.

The Chinatown Plague: Bubonic Plague, San Francisco, 1900
Bibel, D.J., and Chen, T.H. "Diagnosis of Plaque: An Analysis of the Yersin-Kitasato Controversy." 1976. *Bacteriology Review* 40 (3): 633–651.

Markel, Howard. *When Germs Travel*. 2004. New York: Pantheon Books.

Down by the Riverside: Sleeping Sickness, Uganda, 1901
Koerner, T., P. de Raadt, and I. Maudlin. "The 1901 Uganda Sleeping Sickness Epidemic Revisited: A Case of Mistaken Identity?" 1995. *Parasitology Today* 11 (8): 303–306. doi. org/10.1016/0169-4758(95)80046-8.

Steverding, Dietmar. "The History of African Trypanosomiasis." 2008. *Parasites and Vectors* 1 (1): 3. http://dx.doi.org/ doi:10.1186/1756-3305-1-3.

Typhoid Mary and Friends: Typhoid Fever, New York, 1907
Leavitt, Judith Walzer. *Typhoid Mary*. 1996. Boston: Beacon Press.

Bourdain, Anthony. *Typhoid Mary: An Urban Historical*. 2001. London: Bloomsbury.

Soper, George A. "The Work of a Chronic Typhoid Germ Distributor." 1907. *JAMA* XLVIII (24): 2019. http://dx.doi.org/ doi:10.1001/jama.1907.25220500025002d.

An Unpopular Discovery: Pellagra, Mississippi, 1914
Rajakumar, Kumaravel. "Pellagra in the United States." 2000. *Southern Medical Journal* 93 (3): 272–277. http://dx.doi.org/ doi:10.1097/00007611-200093030-00005.

The "Spanish" Flu: Influenza, Worldwide, 1918

Davis, Ryan A. *The Spanish Flu: Narrative and Cultural Identity in Spain, 1918*. 2013. New York: Palgrave Macmillan.

Morens, David M., and Anthony S. Fauci. "The 1918 Influenza Pandemic: Insights for the 21st Century." 2007. *Journal of Infectious Diseases* 195 (7): 1018–1028. http://dx.doi.org/doi:10.1086/511989.

Serum by Dogsled: Diphtheria, Alaska, 1925

Markel, Howard. "Long Ago Against Diphtheria, the Heroes Were Horses," July 10, 2007. *New York Times*.

Salisbury, Gay, and Laney Salisbury. *The Cruelest Miles: The Heroic Story of Dogs and Men in a Race Against an Epidemic*. 2003. New York: W.W. Norton & Co.

Just Another Horror: Typhus, Poland, 1945

Allen, Arthur. *The Fantastic Laboratory of Dr. Weigl: How Two Brave Scientists Battled Typhus and Sabotaged the Nazis*. 2015. New York: W.W. Norton & Co.

Zinsser, Hans. *Rats, Lice and History: A Chronicle of Pestilence and Plagues*. 1935. New York: Black Dog.

The Beginning of the End for Polio: Polio, USA, 1952

Oshinsky, David M. *Polio: An American Story*. 2005. Oxford: Oxford University Press.

Smith, Jane S. *Patenting the Sun*. 1990. New York: W. Morrow.

Breakbone Fever: Dengue, Hemorrhagic Fever, Philippines, 1953

Gubler, D.J., and Goro Kuno. *Dengue and Dengue Hemorrhagic Fever*. 1997. Wallingford, Oxon, UK: CAB International.

The Brain-Eating Amoeba: Primary Amebic Meningoencephalitis, Australia, 1965

Carter, R.F. "Primary Amoebic Meningo-Encephalitis: Clinical, Pathological and Epidemiological Features of Six Fatal Cases." 1968. *J. Pathol.* 96 (1): 1–25. http://dx.doi.org/doi:10.1002/path.1700960102.

De Jonckheere, Johan F. "What Do We Know By Now About the Genus *Naegleria?*" 2014. *Experimental Parasitology* 145: S2-S9. http://dx.doi.org/doi:10.1016/j.exppara.2014.07.011.

The Leak from Compound 19: Anthrax, USSR, 1979
Guillemin, Jeanne. *Anthrax: The Investigation of a Deadly Outbreak.* 1999. Berkeley: University of California Press.

AIDS Panic and Progress: AIDS, USA, 1980s
Giblin, James, and David Frampton. *When Plague Strikes.* 1995. New York: HarperCollins.

Shilts, Randy. *And the Band Played On.* 1987. New York: St. Martin's Press.

Whiteside, Alan. *HIV/AIDS: A Very Short Introduction.* 2008. Oxford: Oxford University Press.

Mad Cow Spreads to Humans: Transmissible Spongiform Encephalopathy, England, 1996
Schwartz, Maxime. *How the Cows Turned Mad: Unlocking the Mysteries of Mad Cow Disease.* 2003. Berkeley: University of California Press.

The Locker Room Menace: MRSA, Los Angeles, 2002
McKenna, Maryn. *Superbug: The Fatal Menace of MRSA.* 2010. New York: Free Press.

The Secret Epidemic: SARS, Hong Kong, 2003
Abraham, Thomas. *Twenty-First Century Plague.* 2005. Baltimore: Johns Hopkins University Press.

Greenfeld, Karl Taro. *China Syndrome.* 2006. New York: HarperCollins.

Ebola Is Real: Ebola, West Africa, 2014
Stern, Jeffrey E. "Hell in the Hot Zone." *Vanity Fair,* October 2014. www.vanityfair.com/news/2014/10/ebola-virus-epidemic-containment.

Quammen, David. *Ebola.* 2014. New York: W.W. Norton.

INDEX

Africa
   Ebola (West Africa), 236–41
   malaria epidemic, 9–12
   schistosomiasis (Egypt), 114–17
   scurvy (Egypt), 45–48
   sleeping sickness (Uganda),
      169–72
AIDS panic and progress (USA),
   216–20
Alaska, diphtheria outbreak, 187–91
Americas. See also Hawaii
   AIDS panic and progress (USA),
      216–20
   bubonic plague (Chinatown, San
      Francisco), 164–68
   diphtheria outbreak (Alaska),
      187–91
   flu epidemic (Hispaniola/Haiti),
      68–71
   influenza (Hispaniola/Haiti),
      68–71
   malaria miracle cure (Peru),
      99–103
   MRSA (Los Angeles), 227–30
   pellagra epidemic (Mississippi),
      178–82
   polio (USA), 197–201
   scurvy (Stadacona/Quebec),
      86–89
   smallpox (Tenochtitlán, Mexico),
      82–85
   Typhoid Mary (New York),
      173–77
   unknown disease
      (Massachusetts), 94–98
   yellow fever (Haiti), 123–26
   yellow fever (Philadelphia),
      109–13
Amoeba, brain-eating, 207–10

Anemia, miner's. See Hookworms
   (Switzerland)
Anthony, Saint, fire of (ergotism),
   41–44
Anthrax outbreak (USSR), 211–15
Asia
   beriberi and thiamin deficiency
      (Japan), 159–63
   bubonic plague (China), 54–58
   cholera pandemic origins (India),
      127–30
   dengue hemorrhagic (breakbone)
      fever (Philippines), 202–6
   measles epidemic (Fiji), 145–49
   SARS (Hong Kong), 231–35
   smallpox epidemic (China),
      37–40
   smallpox epidemic (Japan),
      32–36
Athens, plague of, 18–22
Australia, primary amebic meningo-
   encephalitis, 207–10

Baker, Dr. Sara Josephine, 175
Beriberi (Japan), 159–63
Bilharz, Theodor, 116
"Black Death." See Bubonic plague
Blood, hemorrhaging. See Dengue
   hemorrhagic fever
Bloodletting, 25–26, 40, 62, 111,
   112, 130, 160
Brain-eating amoeba (Australia),
   207–10
Breakbone fever (Philippines),
   202–6
Bubonic plague
   about: facts summaries, 28, 54,
      59, 104, 164
   astrological predictions, 63

Bubonic plague—*continued*
  as "Black Death," 60
  in China (C. 1331), 54–58
  conditions giving rise to, 30–31
  in Europe (1348), 59–63
  in Europe (1665, London), 104–8
  fire, soap and, 107–8
  first appearance, 29
  flagellants and, 61, 62
  footprints in China, 57–58
  futility of treating, 62–63
  germ discovered, 166
  impact of, 29
  origins/carriers and evolution,
      29–30, 55–57, 107–8,
      165–66, 167–68
  other rodent carriers, 56
  plague of Athens and, 19, 21, 22
  Plague of Justinian (C.E. 542,
      Constantinople), 28–31
  Rats, rat fleas and, 30–31, 56–57,
      107–8, 165, 166, 167–68
  religious fears and scapegoats,
      61–62
  in San Francisco (1900,
      Chinatown), 164–68
  tarbagans and, 55
  traveling and spreading, 56–58

Caius, John, 65, 66
Cakobau, Seru Epinisa, 146–47
Cartier, Jacques, 87
Childbed fever (Vienna), 131–35
China
  bubonic plague, 54–58
  SARS (Hong Kong), 231–35
  smallpox epidemic, 37–40
Cholera
  about: facts summaries, 127, 136
  fertile habitat for, 128–29
  in London (1854), 136–40
  mapping leading to cause of,
      138–40
  origins and cause, 128–29, 137–40
  pandemic origins (India), 127–30
  spreading of, 129–30
  treating, 130
CJD (Creutzfeldt-Jakob disease),
    224–25
Constantinople, bubonic plague,
    28–31
Consumption. *See* Tuberculosis
Cortés, Hernan, 83–84, 85
Creutzfeldt-Jakob disease (CJD),
    224–25
Crusades, leprosy and, 49–53
Crusades, scurvy and, 45–48
Cuitláhuac, 84–85

Dancing plague, 77–81
Dengue hemorrhagic fever
    (Philippines), 202–6
Diphtheria outbreak (Alaska),
    187–91
DNA
  of bubonic plague bacterium, 60
  of cholera bacterium, 129
  CJD and, 224
  HIV and, 219
  leprosy analysis, 51
  malaria and, 11–12
  MRSA analysis, 228, 229
  plague of Athens analysis, 21–22
  of "Spanish" flu virus, 185
Dogsleds, delivering diphtheria
    serum, 189–90

Ebola, in West Africa, 236–41
Ebola, plague of Athens and, 21–22
Egypt, scurvy in, 45–48
England
  bubonic plague (London), 104–8
  cholera (London), 136–40
  mad cow disease, 221–26
  sweating sickness, 64–67
  tuberculosis, 118–22

Ergotism (France), 41–44
Europe
  anthrax outbreak (USSR), 211–15
  bubonic plague, 59–63, 104–8
  childbed fever, uterine infection
    (Vienna), 131–35
  cholera (London), 136–40
  dancing plague (Strasbourg),
    77–81
  ergotism (France), 41–44
  Galen's plague (Rome), 23–27
  hookworms (Switzerland),
    150–54
  leprosy and Knights of Lazarus,
    49–53
  mad cow disease (England),
    221–26
  plague of Athens, 18–22
  rabies conquered (Paris), 155–58
  scrofula (France), 90–93
  sweating sickness (England),
    64–67
  syphilis (Italy), 72–76
  tuberculosis (England), 118–22
  typhus epidemic (Poland),
    192–96

Facemasks, SARS and, 232–34
Fever. See also Malaria; Yellow fever
  childbed, uterine infection,
    131–35
  dengue hemorrhagic/breakbone,
    202–6
  Indian, 97–98
  snail, 116–17
  sweating sickness and, 64–67
  unknown disease
    (Massachusetts), 94–98
Fiery serpent (Guinea worm), 13–17
Fiji, measles epidemic, 145–49
Fire, of Saint Anthony, 41–44
"Flesh eating" bacterial infection,
  228

Flu. See Influenza
France
  ergotism, 41–44
  rabies conquered, 155–58
  scrofula, 90–93
French disease. See Syphilis

Galen's plague (Rome), 23–27
Guinea worm (Red Sea), 13–17

Haiti, flu epidemic, 68–71
Haiti, yellow fever epidemic,
  123–26
Hamilton, Alexander, 110, 111
Hansen's disease. See Leprosy
Hantavirus, 67
Hawaii, leprosy on Molokai, 141–44
Hemorrhagic fever, 202–6
Hispaniola/Haiti flu epidemic, 68–71
HIV/AIDS panic and progress (USA),
  216–20
Hong Kong, SARS, 231–35
Hookworms (Switzerland), 150–54
Hookworms, pellagra and, 179
Hutten, Ulrich von, 73, 74, 75

India, cholera pandemic origins,
  127–30
Indian fever, 97–98
Influenza
  about: facts summaries, 68, 183
  bird flu, 185, 233
  Hispaniola/Haiti epidemic, 68–71
  HLA proteins and, 70
  H1N1, 186
  killing healthy young adults, 185
  origins and cause, 185–86
  "Spanish" flu (worldwide), 183–86
  swine flu, 70–71
  virus characteristics and, 69–70,
    185–86
  viruses combining to create,
    185–86

Italy, Galen's plague, 23–27
Italy, syphilis outbreak, 72–76

Japan
    beriberi and thiamin deficiency, 159–63
    impact of epidemics, 33
    smallpox epidemic, 32–36
Justinian, plague of (Constantinople), 28–31

King's evil (scrofula), 90–93
Kitasato, Shibasaburo, 166, 168
Knights of Lazarus, 49–53
Koch, Dr. Robert, 121, 223
Kuru, 223–24

Leprosy
    about: facts summaries, 49, 141
    contagiousness of, 50–51, 142
    criminalization of and exile for, 141–44
    decline and fall of, 51–53
    as Hansen's disease, 50
    Knights of Lazarus and, 49–53
    on Molokai (Hawaii), 141–44
    mystery of, 52–53
    treating, 143–44
    tuberculosis and, 52
Leptospirosis, 97–98
Lice, typhus and, 192–96
Lind, James, 88, 89
Locker room menace, MRSA (Los Angeles), 227–30
London. See England
L'Ouverture, Toussaint, 124, 126
LSD, ergotism and, 44

Mad cow disease (England), 221–26
Malaria
    about: facts summaries, 9, 99
    Africa epidemic, 9–12
    biochemistry of, 10–11

cause of, 9, 12, 100
    DNA, genetics and, 11–12
    early writings on, 10
    first miracle cure, 99–103
    in Peru, 99–103
Mallon, Mary (Typhoid Mary), 173–77
Mass psychogenic illness, 77–81
Measles, plague of Athens and, 21, 22
Measles epidemic (Fiji), 145–49
Mexico (Tenochtitlán), smallpox outbreak, 82–85
Miner's anemia. See Hookworms (Switzerland)
Mississippi, pellagra epidemic, 178–82
Moctezuma, smallpox and, 84–85
Molokai, leprosy on, 141–44
Montagu, Lady Mary Wortley, 39–40
Mosquito-borne diseases. See Dengue hemorrhagic fever; Malaria; Yellow fever
MRSA (Los Angeles), 227–30
Mushers, delivering diphtheria serum, 189–90

Necrotizing fasciitis, 228
New World. See Americas
New York, Typhoid Mary, 173–77
Nutrition-based illnesses
    beriberi and thiamin deficiency (Japan), 159–63
    pellagra and niacin deficiency (Mississippi), 178–82
    vitamin C deficiency. See Scurvy

Pasteur, Louis, 156–58, 223
Peeing red (schistosomiasis), 114–17
Pellagra epidemic (Mississippi), 178–82

Philippines, dengue hemorrhagic (breakbone) fever, 202–6
Plagues. *See also* Bubonic plague
   about: historical overview, 7–8
   of Athens, 18–22
   of children, 189–90
   dancing, 77–81
   of Galen (Rome), 23–27
   of Justinian (Constantinople), 28–31
Poland, typhus epidemic, 192–96
Polio (USA), 197–201
Primary amebic meningo-encephalitis (Australia), 207–10
Procopius, 29–30, 31, 55
Psychogenic illness, mass, 77–81

Rabies conquered (Paris), 155–58
Rats and rat fleas. *See* Bubonic plague
Rats/rat fleas, bubonic plague and, 30–31
Reading, further, 242–50
Red sea, guinea worm (Red Sea), 13–17
RNA, plague of Athens and, 22
Romantic disease. *See* Tuberculosis
Rush, Dr. Benjamin, 11–12

Sabin, Albert, 198, 201
Saint Anthony's fire (ergotism), 41–44
Saint-Domingue (Haiti), yellow fever, 123–26
Salk, Jonas, 198, 201
SARS (Hong Kong), 231–35
Schistosomiasis (Egypt), 114–17
Scrapie. *See* Mad cow disease
Scrofula, 90–93
Scurvy
   about: facts summaries, 45, 86
   cure found and lost, 87–88
   discovering cause of, 88, 89

   doomed crusade (Egypt) and, 45–48
   in Stadacona (Quebec), 86–89
   today, 48
   vitamin C and, 47–48, 87, 88, 89
Secret epidemic (SARS), 231–35
Semmelweis, Ignaz, 132, 133–34
Sleeping sickness (Uganda), 169–72
Smallpox
   about: facts summaries, 23, 32, 37, 82
   in China, 37–40
   Galen's plague (Rome), 23–27
   inoculations for, 38–40
   in Japan, 32–36
   Moctezuma and, 84–85
   mortality rate, 33
   plague of Athens and, 21
   symptoms, 33–34
   in Tenochtitlán (Mexico), 82–85
   treating, 34–35, 38–40
   treatment protocol of Galen and, 24–26
Snail fever, 116–17
Snow, John, 137, 138–40
Soper, George, 174–75
Soviet Union, anthrax outbreak, 211–15
"Spanish" flu (worldwide), 183–86
Squanto's backstory (Massachusetts), 94–98
Strasbourg, dancing plague and, 77–81
Sweating sickness (England), 64–67
Swine flu, 70–71
Switzerland, hookworms, 150–54
Syphilis, 11, 72–76, 87, 115, 142

Takaki, Kanehiro, 160–62
Tenochtitlán, smallpox outbreak, 82–85
Thiamin deficiency, beriberi and, 159–63

Thucydides, 19, 20–21
Transmissible spongiform
  encephalopathy (England),
  221–26
Treating diseases. *See also specific*
  diseases
  four humors and, 25, 39, 62, 66,
    74, 130, 132
  Galen's impact on, 24–26
  inoculations for, 38–40
Tuberculosis
  contagiousness of, 119–21, 122
  in England, 118–22
  king's touch and, 91–93
  leprosy and, 52
  lymph nodes and, 92, 120
  remedy, 121–22
  scrofula (France), 90–93
  as "white plague," 119
Typhoid fever
  contagiousness of, 176–77
  healthy carriers, 176–77
  identifying source of, 174–75
  plague of Athens and, 21–22
  Typhoid Mary (New York), 173–77
Typhus epidemic (Poland), 192–96

Uganda, sleeping sickness, 169–72
United States of America. *See also*
  Hawaii
  AIDS panic and progress, 216–20
  bubonic plague (Chinatown, San
    Francisco), 164–68
  diphtheria outbreak (Alaska),
    187–91
  MRSA (Los Angeles), 227–30
  pellagra epidemic (Mississippi),
    178–82
  polio (USA), 197–201
  Squanto's backstory
    (Massachusetts), 94–98
  Typhoid Mary (New York), 173–77

yellow fever (Philadelphia),
  109–13
Unknown diseases
  plague of Athens, 18–22
  Squanto's backstory
    (Massachusetts), 94–98
  sweating sickness (England),
    64–67
Urine disease. *See* Schistosomiasis
  (Egypt)
USSR, anthrax outbreak, 211–15
Uterine infection (Vienna), 131–35

Vienna, childbed fever (uterine
  infection), 131–35
Virus, term origin, 156
Vitamin B deficiencies
  beriberi (Japan), 159–63
  pellagra (Mississippi), 178–82
Vitamin C lack. *See* Scurvy

Welch, Dr. Curtis, 188, 189, 190
West Africa, Ebola, 236–41
Whitehead, Rev. Henry, 137, 140
World War II
  dengue hemorrhagic fever and,
    202–6
  pellagra problem and, 182
  typhus epidemic (Poland),
    192–96

Yaws, 11, 76
Yellow fever
  about: facts summaries, 109, 123
  African Americans and, 112–13
  cause of, 125–26
  in Haiti, 123–26
  in Philadelphia, 109–13
  treating, 110–12
Yersin, Alexandre, 166, 168. *See*
  also Bubonic plague